GYMNASTIC EDUCATION

Count Fritz von Bothmer

Translated with an Introduction by Olive Whicher

MERCURY PRESS

ISBN 978-1-957569-50-5

Published by
MERCURY PRE SS
an imprint of SteinerBooks
PO Box 58
Hudson, New York 12534
www.steinerbooks.org

CONTENTS

Foreword

Fritz Graf von Bothmer developed gymnastic exercises in the 1920s for the children of the first Waldorf School at the request of Dr. Rudolf Steiner, who was one of the founders of the school. This was to teach posture and to develop movements in the children's limbs, which would augment pedagogy. He developed approximately thirty exercises. They are a study of the archetypal dynamics of the human being in space.

Fritz Graf von Bothmer taught gymnastics at the Stuttgart Waldorf School in Germany until 1938 when this school was closed by the regime in Germany at the time. Movement was being restricted on many levels. In the three years following the school closing he wrote down his experiences gained from working with the children. When he died in 1941 this book was complete. Originally there were no pictures accompanying the descriptions. His friend and the original editor of this book, Gisbert Husemann, M.D., found photographs in Bothmer's estate of his exercise demonstrations and added them to the text. Elizabeth and Wolfgang Dessecker, pupils of Bothmer, edited the text, gave musical examples and completed the photographic presentation of the exercises. Thanks to the work of Olive Whicher part of this text has been available in English since 1959. Gisbert Husemann was instrumental in publishing this book again in English. Jaimen McMillan retranslated Bothmer's original text.

Until recently the Bothmer gymnastics exercises were practiced mainly in the domain of Waldorf classes. With the increase in activity brought about by Jaimen McMillan's spatial dynamics training, interest in the original Bothmer manuscript evolved.

It is difficult to show movement or to demonstrate the actual gestures by photographs. To do the exercises correctly the gymnast must maintain proper balance of "threefold man" (nerve-sense, rhythmic and metabolic-limb) in all planes. This is the picture of health. A correct practice can bring about healing of body and soul. What is so needed in education and practice today is free conscious will activity. Until recently Bothmer gymnastics was one of the least known of therapeutic modalities available to physicians.

Many teachers and medical professionals who have completed the training are now teaching spatial dynamics and Bothmer gym to schoolchildren and patients. Children and adults today on the whole move less and many have developmental movement problems. The relationship between impaired movement and school performance has long been established, stressing the importance of developing fine and gross motor coordination in the growing child. Bothmer gym helps the children of today, who often grow up without the opportunity to participate in physical play and games, to find freedom in their movement again. Children and adults whose senses and nervous system are over stimulated can reconnect to their rhythmic middle system and active will in the limbs. This therapeutic modality is distinct from therapeutic eurythmy and often a patient can be working on both forms of movement.

A beautiful and truthful movement flows from point to infinity. Its origins are in infinity. As Bothmer tells us: "the goal is to use the play of forces at work in human movement in such a way as to evoke the ideal picture of greater man living in space."

May this edition of Bothmer's book further study and practice of the free movement of the human being in space.

These exercises are taught at the *Bothmer Schule for Gymnastik* in Stuttgart, Germany and throughout the world as part of the five year Spatial Dynamics training. Information can be obtained from the Spatial Studies Institute, Inc., 423 Route 71, Hillside, N.Y. 12529. Phone and Fax (518) 325-7096.

Joan Takacs, D.O. and Christa van Heek van Tellingen, M.D.

Translator's Preface

This volume contains the translation into English of the two main parts of the book *Gymastische Erziehung* in which the manuscript left by Count Fritz von Bothmer when he died in 1941 has been published for the first time, under the auspices of the Pedagogical Section of the Goetheanum, Dornach, Switzerland and under the editorship of Gisbert Husemann M.D. of Stuttgart. Preceding it is the Introductory chapter by the present writer.

Count Bothmer was among the group of teachers called together by Rudolf Steiner in the early years of the Waldorf School, Stuttgart, to develop new educational methods in accordance with a modern spiritual conception of the nature of man. Physical education was Bothmer's task. The manuscript, entitled Gymnastic Education, embodied the attempt he made to put into words his basically new approach to this task and to set down the complete sequence of gymnastic exercises created during many years of work with the children. This writing was a difficult task; for as he so often said, it is only in doing the exercises that one really learns to know and appreciate them.

Count Bothmer left an incomplete set of drawings - very beautiful but impossible to reproduce - and the volume of illustrations accompanying this book, compiled with the help of Mr. and Mrs. Wolfgang Dessecker, Stuttgart, has been based partly on these and partly on photographs, some taken with Mrs. Dessecker's co-operation and others, early ones, showing the teacher himself at work. Elisabeth Dessecker, who was one of Bothmer's leading pupils, has also annotated the text and added the curriculum, all of which should greatly help the reader to follow and understand the sequence of movements in the exercises. The latter cover a period of twelve school years, the children advancing in the sequence as they grow through the school. In Bothmer's words, "each exercise is a whole, a movement picture into which the child can grow."

The chapter on Human Movement in Physical and Ethereal Space makes fruitful for gymnastics the new conception of space give by Rudolf Steiner and developed by Mr. George Adams, Prof. Louis Locher and others; it is the outcome of some years' experience in teaching gymnastics in Rudolf Steiner schools.

Bothmer makes wonderfully graphic use of spatial terms to mean quite definite positions and movements of the body, thus using the flexible quality of the German language to describe long sequences of movement in very few words. This spatial language has been adhered to in the translation, although the equivalent English words, not having the same phonetic sound or rhythm, do not always paint the picture of the movement with quite the same color. The illustrations should help the reader to find his way into the exact meaning of these expressions. For example, "Height" (*Höhe*) means both arms raised vertically upward with the whole body poised on the toes. "Width" (*Weite*) means standing on the toes with arms outspread sideways, palms facing upward; while with "breadth" (*Breite*) the feet are full on the ground and palms face down. Bothmer often accompanied the exercises with words or verses, giving at the same time the spatial picture and the rhythm of the movement. This presented a difficulty in translation, and the English teacher may well prefer to create a new world picture himself out of the genius of his own language. It would be well to note that the German word "*Gymnastik*" refers to exercises of the body pure and simple, while a distinct word "*Turnen*" is used for work on the apparatus. It is in the nature of the Bothmer gymnastic exercises that though they are simply bodily exercises, yet they form the basis and leitmotif for all else that is done in the gymnasium during the different stages of child development.

We in the English-speaking world, where Bothmer's work is steadily growing, are grateful to the publishers of *Gymnastische Erziehung* for including this long awaited English translation. Through the efforts of Mr. Knut Ross and the College of Teachers in Michael Hall, Forest Row, Sussex, a growing number of teachers are being trained in the new approach to physical education and are finding their way into Rudolf Steiner Schools in many countries.

Olive Whicher
Goethean Science Foundation
Clent, Worcester, England

Human Movement in Physical and Ethereal Space

Olive Whicher

Count Bothmer's work in gymnastic movement led him to an experience of space going far beyond the rigid, three-dimensional Euclidean conception of space, which dominated scientific thought until very recent times. Bothmer considered that he had come, not through intellectual thought, but through the practice of bodily movement, to an experience of what he called the "forces of space". While he was practicing and developing his gymnastic exercises, which he did long and often, he became aware of the creative, spiritual forces of space which work upon the human body, Rudolf Steiner also spoke of such forces.

It was a fundamental principle of Bothmer's pedagogical striving, to bring to the growing child a real experience of this spiritual quality of space, wherein the ideal picture of man and of his bodily movements is to be found. "Man stands, in the balance of his forces, between gravity, which would draw him downward, and the sphere he bears above his shoulders; he stands upright in the vertical, reaching out and spanned into breadth and width in the horizontal". Space as Bothmer experiences it, is not merely outer form. "Height", "Depth" and "the Horizontal" are also forces. Man is to be in control of the forces which pull him downward and of those which draw him upward; he shall live in the balance between them. Through a kind of gymnastic movement which is in accord with a more living and spiritual conception of how the human being is incarnated into space, the child should learn to live in three, dimensional earthly space, without becoming imprisoned in the physical, material world. Through movement the rigid immobility of this space will be overcome, and space itself will be experienced spiritually once more; man will rise above the merely external, spatial aspect of incarnation and become truly free. Space is in reality threefold, like Man; in gymnastic movement Man reveals Space and Space reveals Man.

It is a different direction from that taken by most modern schools of movement, for they are based upon the one-sidedly physical and mechanical picture of the human body which is popular today. Bothmer underlines the fact that he evolved his exercises as the result of what he calls his "researches into space", - that is to say, in exploring and discovering the way the human being really lives and moves in space. In Gymnastics, he said, the ego strives, via the body, to find its relationship with space, and the practice of gymnastic movement should be determined, not by intellectual reasoning alone, nor by blind instinct, but as a result of research into space. We need to understand the true character of the space in which the body moves. Bothmer regarded gymnastics as pure movement; uncolored by feeling, and he thought that gymnastic movements could only be true and not meaningless if they accorded with a proper understanding of the laws of space. One of the distinguishing features of his work may be expressed in his own words; "If in practicing bodily movement we take our start from research into the laws of space and listen to its clear rhythms, we shall find deep sense and purpose in the resulting movements. We can discover that in our movements space reveals itself as a spiritual process, and that the body, through which we experience space, is itself a part of this process."

To attempt to reach to the depths of what Bothmer tried to describe about bodily movement in space leads to a realization of the inner sense and true pedagogical value of his work - to that in it which is really new. It also avoids the danger of simply copying the form of the exercises and doing them without reference to the deeper, less one-sidedly physical quality of movement they require. The feeling of responsibility grows with practice, as anyone knows who has tried to work seriously in the field. It is the "perceptive insight" into the whole realm of human movement, so stressed by Bothmer, which must be achieved and put to the test; only in this spirit are we justified in taking up his work and developing it further.

Just as Bothmer laid little emphasis on the importance of putting the results of his gymnastic self-training into words, so it is difficult for those who are only familiar with the ideas about space which are derived from classical geometry to understand his attempts at explanation. The truth and significance of what Bothmer struggles to describe is, however, evident to anyone who is imbued with the thoughts about space which have been developed in our time as an outcome of the union of modern Projective Geometry with Spiritual Science. The ideas which slowly dawned upon Bothmer during his intensive activity of will in the development and practice of his exercises may than be formulated clearly, with an exact thinking which reaches beyond the one-sidedly physical conception of space based upon ancient geometry. To do this is essential, for we are concerned with the manner in which man, a cosmic and earthly being, moves in cosmic and earthly space.

Man's experience of the wide circle of the horizon around him, and the heavenly vault above, is in great contrast with the way he feels this earth beneath his feet. Above and around him he receives the light and perceives the world consciously through his sense of sight; below, as though in the darkness, he touches the earth. Standing and walking upon the earth, he is supported by his legs, two strong pillars upon which the weight of his body rests. They do not possess an awakened consciousness; but they are endowed with the power to resist the forces of gravity and to sustain the heavy body. There are, however, other forces concerned in holding the body upright; they function through man's waking consciousness, for when the light of consciousness is dimmed or extinguished, the body falls to the ground. To be able to stand and walk properly, we must be aware of our surroundings. In fact, we hold ourselves upright as much through our sense of sight, which can be directed to the encircling horizon, as through the way our feet tread the earth. (In blindness, other senses play their part in maintaining awareness of the world around.) Earthward is the domain of darkness and weight, above is light and lightness; and man's upright stature depends on the dynamic interplay of polar opposite forces.

This is really where Bothmer takes his start, and in learning his exercises one comes to realize that human movement is a rhythmical outcome of the interplay of the great universal polarities, call them as one will; the Heights and Depths, Levity and Gravity, Light and Darkness, Periphery and Center. It is a truly Goethean conception.

Further, Bothmer recognizes that the child has a changing relationship to the interplay of the forces of gravity and levity during the different stages of his development. He comes to the earth ('von der Weite her' - "Out of the everywhere into here"), endowed with heavenly forces from the worlds of light and gradually meets with the forces of earth. The way through childhood is a process of metamorphosis, and this is revealed in the change in character and quality of the child's movements as he grows older, for his movements are an expression of the way in which the spirit indwells the body. Healthy school gymnastics must be based upon this fact, because the teacher of gymnastics, in calling for gymnastic movement, comes to meet the gradually incarnating ego of the child. The ego is to learn how to live in space.

What then is space? Modern Geometry supplements the classical geometry of Euclid and provides a more complete and spiritual conception of space. Euclid starts from points; the things of the earth are measured; sizes and proportions are in terms of finite lengths, areas, volumes; the quality of the thought is pointwise and the geometry is concerned with finite forms. The straight line is the shortest distance between two points; it is the sum of so many unit lengths. In the limit the line is made up of an infinite number of points. Euclidean Geometry describes relationships between point-centers and accords with the very nature of the physical-material earth. Projective Geometry however recognizes not only the aspect of the point, but also that of the plane. It shows how forms are also created planewise; a form can be conceived ideally in the relationship not only of its point centers, but also of its planes - planes which will often mould it plastically from outside. Both aspects taken together provide laws of space according to which forms in metamorphosis may be studied, - for example, the changing and developing forms of the living kingdoms of nature. This Geometry brings the rigid Euclidean forms into movement; the limited, finite forms pass over into infinite ones. To the points are added the planes, to the straight line as a manifold of points is added the line as a totality and the line membered of all its planes. Between mid-point and infinitely distant plane, forms are created which follow one another rhythmically and in metamorphosis. Even space itself is capable of undergoing a radical metamorphosis. The new geometry opens the way to an understanding of living forms which come into being, develop and pass away again; this happens in the interplay of creative forces which are polar opposite to one another. In the living world, centric and peripheral forces work together, and the result - like an echo of the harmony of the spheres - is rhythm and movement. (1)

Rudolf Steiner often drew attention to the need to gain a new conception of space; he said this was essential, if we would comprehend more fully the kingdom of life and spirit, and he pointed in this connection to the fact that modern projective geometry does already open the way to a more spiritual conception of space. For example, in a course of lectures give in the Hague in April 1922(2), referring to this new geometry, he speaks of a space, - he calls it "Gegenraum", - which is not created centrically, around the three-dimensional axes which meet in a point and ray outward into space, but is formed plastically by planes, from the periphery inward. Then, referring to the ether-body which permeates the physical body of man, he goes on to say, "We can study the physical body if we look within its spatial form for the forces which stream through it. But we cannot learn to know the ether body, - the body of formative forces, - if we remain with our ideas within the spatial form. We can only study the ether body if we realize that planes of force (Kraftflächen) move in towards the earth from all sides and come near to man, plastically molding his body of formative forces from outside."

Here Rudolf Steiner actually speaks of planes of force, which belong originally to the cosmic periphery. In the book "Fundamentals of Therapy", which he wrote together with Dr. Ita Wegman, Rudolf Steiner describes how the formative powers of life, - he calls them the ether-forces or universal forces, - stream in from the world periphery to work counter to the physical laws and imbue a body with life. Without such forces, as a result of which there are substances in the kingdom of earth which are not subject to the physical laws alone but come under the influence of polar opposite laws, a body would lie inert or fall like a stone to the ground. According to the physical laws, says Rudolf Steiner, forces work outward from the earth; the ethereal forces, on the other hand, stream inward towards the earth from all sides of the universe. In describing this, he uses the words "space" and "counterspace" (Raum und Gegenraum); the physical laws and forces are to be found in ordinary space, - the ethereal in a kind of negative space permeating it. Gravity is a physical law; the gravitational force radiates from centers of mass and particularly from the center of the earth. All physical bodies are pulled down by their weight towards the earth's center. Counter to them, the cosmic forces draw upward in the opposite direction; they are upward-bearing forces.

In Projective Geometry, point and plane belong together, they are set over against one another, polar opposite in character, but equal in significance. The ideal point is the extreme picture of contraction; the ideal plane represents the greatest possible expansion. In its totality, the plane extends on all sides without end; it has no edge; and the straight lines which lie in it stretch away into the infinite distances. This polarity of point and plane is fundamental, and it is brought about with respect to the sphere, which derives from the original polarity of point-center and plane-periphery. An active contemplation of Plate 1 will reveal to the thinker that where there is an ideal sphere in space, any movement of planes result in a movement of the points belonging to them; and the converse is also true. Planes moving in from the world periphery towards the sphere will be answered by points which will stream out from the central point within. The sphere itself embodies this latent polarity. It can be formed by many points; the surface and also the interior may consist of an infinite accumulation of points. This would be a sphere in the aspect of density, akin to a heavy body, and its mass would have a convex form. But it is possible to think of a sphere formed by many planes. On all sides, the infinitely many planes (each of which is polar opposite to one of the infinitely many points forming the spherical mass), will envelop and mould the sphere. The planes come in from the cosmic periphery and create the sphere as a hollow form. Now it will not be a dense concentration of points but will be molded plastically from outside, with a hollow spherical space within. The circles in Plate 1 show these form creating processes in a two-dimensional picture. This purely geometrical, precisely scientific concept points to an archetypal phenomenon of creation.

Plate 1

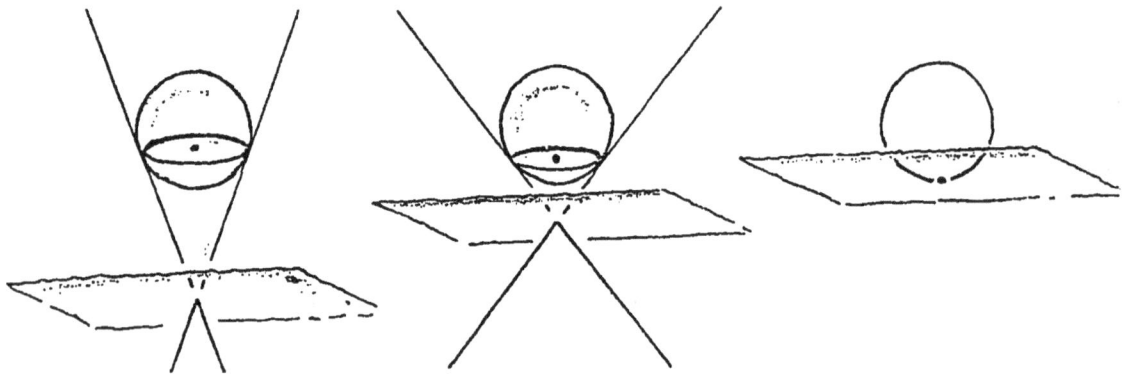

Fig. 1

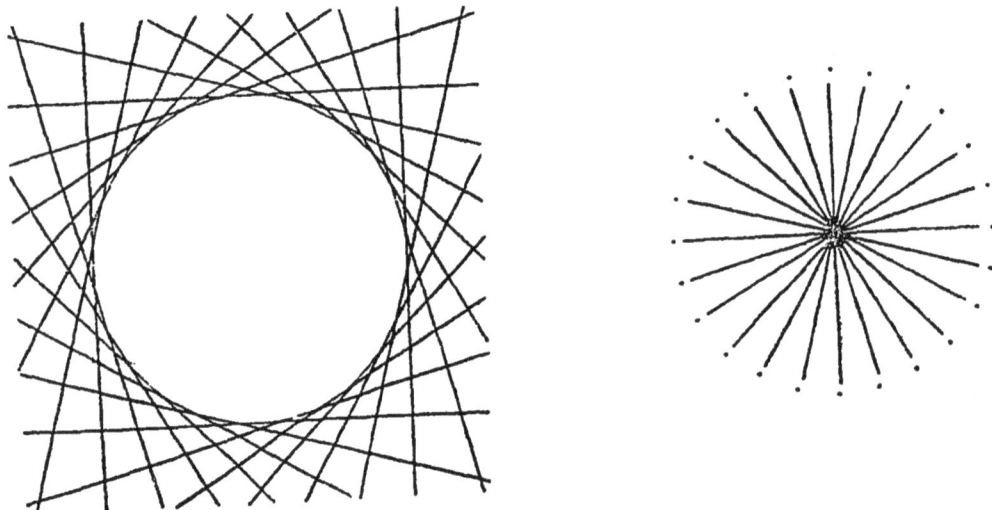

Fig. 2

The pointwise aspect of a ball held in the hand, - a sphere of stone, for example, - is easily comprehended. But the tangent planes enveloping its surface are not necessarily visible, they would have to be added in thought and imagination. To learn to recognize with perceptive insight the ideal planes belonging to any form is of fundamental importance, especially when it is a question of studying living forms. The planes, though they are not usually visible to the senses, may often be perceived immediately in the gesture of the form. Particularly is this so in the plant kingdom. (1) Plant forms, which come into being between Sun and Earth, follow not only the rigid laws of Geo-metry, - the measurement of the forms of earth. They also conform to other laws; laws for which we may use the description Helio-plastic, -moulded by the light-forces of the sun. This holds good for all living and moving forms, where there may be change and metamorphosis, for here the interplay of the great universal polarities is always at work.

The ideal ethereal planes, weaving invisibly about the human being, may actually be perceived in the forms and gestures of his bodily movement; the very signature of the planar forces of the sun may indeed be read in man's movements. In great works of art, too especially in sculpture, though in painting also, it is often striking to see how the planes are at work, plastically moulding the forms. Greek sculptors revealed the ethereal planes in veil and robe and wing, but also in the wonderfully balanced poise of their art. Rudolf Steiner, too, urged that in the plastic arts, forms should be created by the interweaving of planes, and in his art of eurythmy, the forms assumed by the movements of the veil, as it passes through the air, emphasize the plastic and peripheral quality of the arm and hand movements.

There are two main characteristics of the plane: its property of molding forms plastically from without, and that of sustaining an upward bearing force, working contrary to gravity. In both these ways the ethereal plane functions in active contrast to the purely physical laws. In eurythmy, it is perhaps especially the first characteristic which comes to the fore: in Gymnastics the second. This upward-bearing, anti-gravitational quality of movement inherent in the ethereal planes, comes powerfully to expression in the Bothmer Gymnastics, when rightly practiced and understood. While doing the exercises, a true feeling for the upward movement of the ethereal, planes can be awakened, - how they weave in from cosmic infinitudes, surrounding and penetrating the body. The burden of earthly gravity falls from the body and it is endowed with lightness and vitality.

Man alone has arms and hands which do not have to support the body in the gravitational field of earth but are free to be raised towards the sun. The quality and gesture of typical arm and hand movements accords with this fact. A point moves through space with a pointlike, thrusting gesture, like the shot from a gun or a falling stone. But the plane, which moulds plastically, from outside, through its very nature, must move with quite a different gesture; it is an extended entity and therefore it hovers or floats from one position to the next. In the Bothmer exercises, pushing, punching and spear-like arm-movements occur rarely, whereas again and again the arms and hands move in planes. Very often they lie in a plane, and then in moving it is as though the whole plane were moving with them. In these exercises, the arms should never be stretched out stiffly and rigidly from the body; the feeling rather is that they are drawn out and become membered in the hovering planes. It would accord with the true nature of the arms if they were to reach far away out to the horizon - just as far, indeed, as the soul can reach which truly experiences the world. Standing with arms outstretched, one can feel as though an invisible part of the arms were reaching inward from the world-circumference to meet at the fingertips and draw the physical arms outward. In the deeds of his hands, man meets his own destiny; this is the other half of his being, spread out in his environment and coming to meet him at every moment. A healthy feeling of freedom may be experienced as the body stands, with feet firmly on the ground and arms extended in the horizontal plane - in that plane which runs parallel to the ground, passes through the body at about the level of the collar-bone, and extends to the infinitely distant horizon. The plane is experienced livingly, far out beyond the fingertips; physical tension of muscle and bone is diminished and it is as though the arms and hands were actually carried by this plane - upborne by the ether forces and helping to hold the body erect.

We touch here on a vital social element in movement. It is in the realm of this common horizontal plane that men grasp one another by the hand. Two people cannot stand on the same spot in space; their centers of gravity and mass oblige them to be self-centered. But men are united through the cosmic horizon in the great social plane in which their hands meet, - just as children are, who hold hands in a ring. This is the sphere in which the social forces of the heart flow from man to man. It is of the utmost importance to bear this in mind in the development of educational gymnastics.

The hands, and particularly the palms, play an active part in experiencing the plane, and in the Bothmer exercises it almost always makes a difference, which way the palms are facing, whether upward, downward, forward or backward. The palm, held flat, though not rigidly so, is laid into the plane and becomes part of it; thus it becomes a sense organ through which space is experienced. The palm 'sees' into the planar world and part of one's being can flow out through the fingertips into the ethereal infinitudes. It is in the light of such experiences of space that the expressions used by Bothmer, such as "Weite" or "Horizontale" (the Horizontal plane), should be understood. And when Bothmer speaks of the three dimensions, we shall better understand what he really means if we remember that the three-dimensional axes of space are derived from the interpenetration of the three dimensional planes which penetrate the world and the human body spiritually (Plate 2). These geometrical expressions are not meant to be taken statically, but dynamically. The three dimensional planes and the axes in which they interpenetrate, are bearers of the forces of space. (In this picture, the three planes are really to be imagined as extending far away out into space; the circular edges are only added in the picture to make them visible externally.)

Figure 4 is one way of picturing threefold man in the balance of the forces of space. The earthly and cosmic forces interpenetrate; below they are predominantly centric, above they are peripheral (spherical). They meet in the balance of the horizontal. In this balance lives man, "upright in the vertical, spanned into breadth and width in the horizontal".

Plate 2

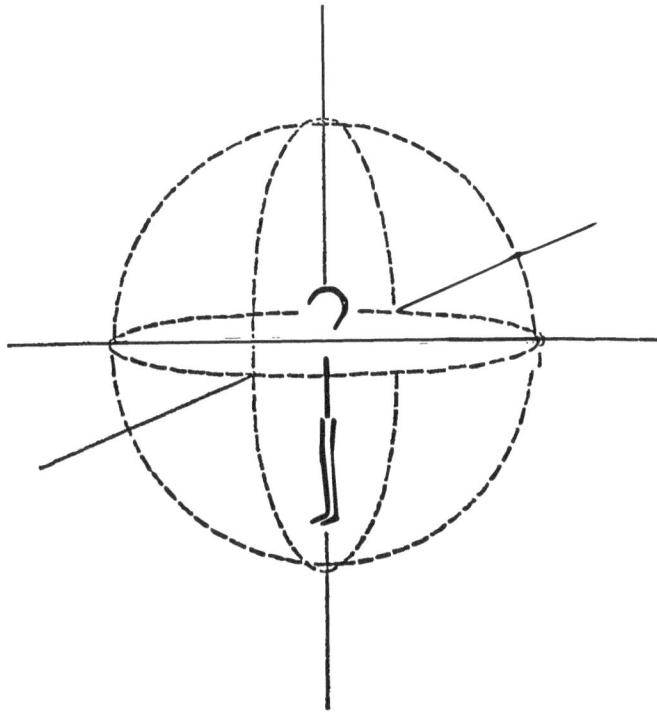

Fig. 3

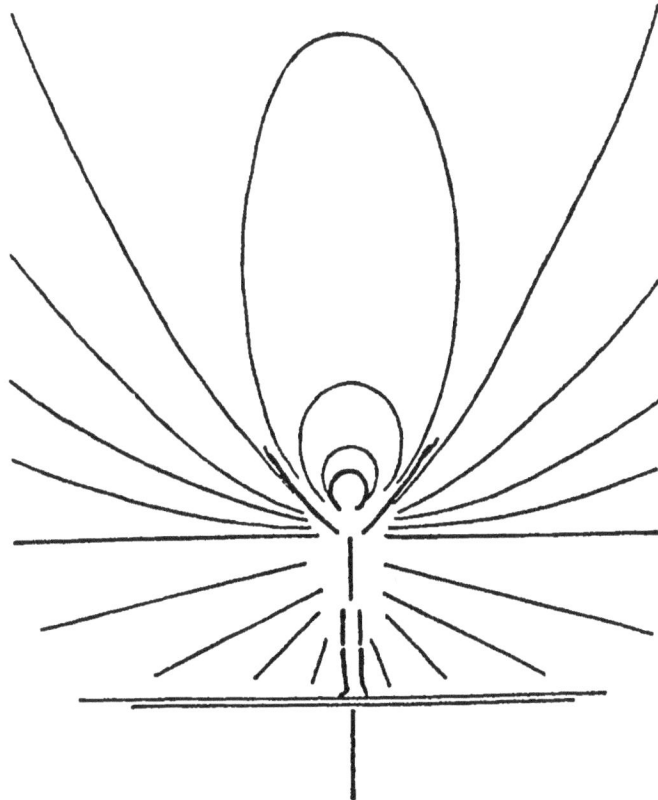

Fig. 4

When, after long practice, the planar forces are really experienced and it becomes clear how greatly the quality of human movement is influenced by an awakened consciousness of these forces, the reality of the ethereal world will dawn for the gymnast. The planes will then no longer be like those of Euclidean geometry, rigid and finite and capable of forming barriers. They will be experienced dynamically and man will be less bound by the material substance and physical weight of his body - he will feel alive!

The healthy human being lives with his ego and his life of feeling in a state of balance between cosmos and earth. Gymnastics and in day-to-day life it is possible to see how a child, particularly before puberty, feels the powers of his body balanced between weight and lightness. The children should enjoy the contrasts in gymnastic movement. How they can stamp upon the ground! And how, on the other hand, they love to climb away from the earth as far as possible and then perhaps to swing, - in some way or other to fly through the air. It is only necessary to watch children at play, jumping and balancing, and see the gesture of their movements, - the ethereal planes are there, and the child has confidence in them. This subconscious feeling for movement which the young child enjoys, should become a conscious experience for the adult. One of the aims of the Bothmer Gymnastics is just this; to preserve for the adult the wonderful confidence in the ethereal, life-sustaining forces which the child brings with him as the gift of life. This confidence must not be lost; the human being must retain it after puberty, but then it will only be his by virtue of powers developed within himself; for puberty means a fall into the depths, and this fall must be surmounted.

*

To watch the miracle of a little child learning to stand and walk is to see him trying to come to terms with two opposite worlds at the same time; that of his own little body, weighed down and held to the spot in the field of earthly gravity, and the world of his environment and the encircling horizon. The child is really endeavoring to bring about a condition of stability and balance between these two. He must first make his legs and feet hold him up, and then he tries, with outstretched arms and hands, to move into his surroundings. What a truth is hidden in the words of the first roundelay, with which Bothmer leads his nine-year-olds into their first gymnastic lessons: "We come from the widths of space". The little child does indeed come from the widths of space and has gradually to find himself in his own center. Surely, too, he is carried at first more by the peripheral forces than by the centric ones. The power which sustains him in his newly found upright position is not the force of gravity; it comes from his environment, his consciousness, from around and above him, - quite another kind of force. And when he falls, what a fall it can be! The little form lies abandoned on the ground, as though the strings of a marionette had snapped, and he waits for someone in his surroundings to put him on his feet again. In this business of learning to walk, the child shows incredible confidence. How often do we not feel that a guardian angel must be near when the child takes his first steps. This feeling could be expressed in the following words. In the first years of life the child is sustained in movement and posture by the starry forces of the universe, - by divine powers. It is the Hands of God, woven into the up-bearing ether-forces surrounding the child, which draw and hold him upright, - the cosmic "planes of force" of the infinite universe!

The human being standing, can be likened to a top, which has an axis in its midst and over against this a horizon. When the top spins, a state of equilibrium is being maintained between axis and circumference. When, while spinning, the top "goes to sleep", it is resting in its own vertical axis; but the world horizon plays an equally important part in this phenomenon. So it is with man. Learning to stand upright means learning to come to rest in one's own vertical axis, - but also in the cosmic periphery. (Of interest in this connection is the fact that in cases of mental disturbance revolving movements often occur.) Every human being who can stand and walk, has found his own vertical axis, like a spiritual staff within him; and he also experiences his horizon. These two belong intimately together.

Though to describe it in detail would go beyond our present scope, modern geometry gives clear definition to the "geometrical and helioplastic" thought-pictures by means of which we recognize the mutual and polar relation of the vertical axis within, and the infinite circle in the plane of the horizon. This is another geometrical picture attainable by clear thinking, which illustrates the great interrelated polarities, between which threefold man has to find his balance. He looks outward into distant infinitudes towards the cosmic horizon which he can never reach physically. But within him too there is the inexhaustible world of his own being, an infinitude within. These two create a polarity and at the same time a unity. The "spiritual staff" within and the world of the "encircling round" answer to one another, around and about them the forces of the Depths pull downward and those of the Heights draw upward. Rudolf Steiner speaks sometimes of this vertical axis and calls it the line of the ego (Ich-linie). "My Vertical" (*Meine Aufrechte*), says Bothmer to the children.

Gradually, in the course of his development, man comes to regard his "Vertical" as something belonging to his own individuality. Descending out of the worlds of light, he comes into the darkness of Earth and meets with the forces of gravity. He must then learn to find within himself the power of the Spirit Light and let it shine like a torch in the darkness until he carries it forth again into the Heights. The human being is deserted by the divine world in order that he may himself give birth to divine forces in the darkness of the Earth. In this lies man's freedom. He finds the powers of upright stature within himself. But it is not physical staff to which he shall be fettered, neither the cold intellect, nor the earthly aspect of the body. "My Vertical" shall not lead to the rigid backbone of a soldier. The spiritual staff within is no despotic power or outward ruling force; it is the bearer of a living, growing process of unfolding and its forces must again and again be renewed through an inner activity of the individual. The body becomes the temple of the human ego, and for the ego to live freely in the temple, a true balance must be maintained between the heights and the depths; there must be harmony between thinking, feeling and willing, - harmony actively created. Bothmer thought it was the task of physical education to serve this unfolding process. To quote his own words again: "We can discover that in our movements space reveals itself as a spiritual process, and that the body, through which we experience space, is itself a part of this process."

*

In the second seven-year period comes the wonderful time when the child is harmoniously balanced between Heaven and Earth. With what lightness of control and agility a child of nine or ten years runs and jumps and climbs. His movements show his command over the earth forces, but it is clear that this happens instinctively rather than consciously. The gymnastics teacher knows well that with children at this age he can rely on an instinctive sureness of movement which he will not necessarily expect of the same children later on. For there comes a time of metamorphosis, - the period of puberty, - when difficulties may arise. The child becomes more conscious of his body, it may feel foreign to him and heavy. The body no longer leaves him free; it is as though his wings are clipped and he is caught. The Light-being of man enters deep into the body; the individuality will have to come to terms with the rigid force of the skeleton. The child's world is shaken.

Unhappily, it is not impossible, particularly in modern times, for the true human being to go astray at this stage in his development, and lose his way in the physical, earthly realm. Much depends upon what kind of treatment the temple of the body has received before and during these years. If only physical laws and concepts dominate the minds of those who care for children, stone walls will be built and the spirit shut either in or out. We are only too familiar with the problem caused by dead thinking and perverted morality in the world today. Among all the subjects taught in a Rudolf Steiner School, the Bothmer Gymnastics can be a powerful force for good. During their earlier years, the children will have lived their way through those exercises characterized by Bothmer as a "Play between Lightness and Weight". Their instinctive confidence in the cosmic planes will have been maintained, not by words but by an activity of will, during the time in which they have been descending deeper and deeper into the realm of earth. Then follows that important exercise, with its many variations, which Bothmer called the "Fall into the Inclined Plane" or "The Fall into Space".

Considered in the light of our present thoughts, this exercise no longer represents an easy "play" between heights and depths. It demands a serious attempt to learn to recognize and know both the peripheral and the centric forces at work in movement. The exercise comprises a fall, not yet into the depths of the pointwise world, but into a particular plane, a plane determined by the individual. Now the power of the ethereal planes is to be put to the test! This exercise is brought to a class just at the time when the child's world begins to crumble but before he has really lost his wings. The divine powers are still sustaining the children in their movement, and yet there is a premonition of a new phase to come, for life begins to demand a greater independence. Much can be achieved educationally through this exercise, if the teacher really does experience the sustaining, uplifting power of the ethereal planes. In Bothmer's words: "This exercise gives a freedom of balance and equilibrium no longer subject to the fixed dimensions of space, but determined by the human form itself". To the children at this stage he gave the words: "I stand upright, firmly on the ground, one foot ready to step forward."

After this Bothmer brings the exercise which he calls "Fall into the Point". For man falls from the wonderful sun-world of childhood-being, woven through with the planes of light, into the narrow, concentrated world of the center of gravity of the Earth. It is the fall into the space in which the Cross is erected.

There then follow the many exercises at which the children also work during the years of adolescence, like the "Fall into the Point", which are so designed that through movement itself the powers of the depths are experienced and surmounted. Will-power, irradiated and sustained by consciousness, meets and overcomes the inertia of the physical body; cosmic, peripheral forces are given spatial and rhythmical form and expression in the gymnastic movements, and Bothmer now says: "Freedom to look and move towards the goal has been achieved".

The young gymnast experiences his humanity in space, - in a space permeated by living creative forces. Even the layman, watching these exercises, quickly recognizes the pure wonder of the spatial forms revealed in the moving human body, and he who looks on with eyes to perceive the ethereal planes, sees how they light forth in the movements, sustaining them. To the young scholars during these years Bothmer said: "I stand upright, firmly on the ground, conscious of the dimensions of space and of the forces which come from its enveloping sphere". Another of his sayings at this time was: "The dimensions of space, which interpenetrate one another and me, I let live in my consciousness as forces of will. I stand".

It is not out of place to think here of the forces of Resurrection, for these are indeed the forces to which Bothmer is reaching in his experience and conception of human movement. Rudolf Steiner once said that in gymnastics the teacher meets with the ego of the child face to face and is able to work upon the ego through the physical body. True, the ego is not yet really within the physical body of the child, but the whole process of development through childhood and adolescence is a preparation for its entry; the rhythms and periods of later life are mirrored in these early years. In normal healthy development a state of equilibrium is again achieved after puberty, the character of which is however quite different from the childlike balance of the nine- or ten-year old. A young girl of seventeen or eighteen may show a grace and poise and also a power in her deportment, which reveals the ego already shining through; noble forces of control and balance are like a promise of what is to come. The adolescent youth goes his way with springing gait, conscious of his aims; he is capable of fortitude, ready and willing to test his strength and his powers of endurance. The forces of thinking have become free and may now enter harmoniously into the life of will. It is the time when the idealism of youth awakens. The young individual looks towards the horizon and prepares to seek out the paths of his destiny among those of his contemporaries in the social life.

At twenty-one, the mature human being goes his further way into life. His development, having come to a certain physical completion, continues now in other ways. Life will still bring tests and probations in the periods to come, but what has been achieved in these early years will remain as a sound foundation. The light of the ego-being may shine far into the world and the world will respond. Bothmer puts it simply when he speaks of the "greater man" who will rise above the dead picture of the three-dimensional world. "The essential task of this school of gymnastics is to allow a greater man to arise in infinite space through the play of forces in human movement, and to see that the finite human body grows more and more into this ideal picture of man, becoming formed and orientated according to it."

*

In the above mentioned lecture at the Hague in 1922, Rudolf Steiner describes how it was the inner meaning of modern Projective Geometry which first caused him to realize the real difference between supersensible and natural vision. For, as he said, in the new geometry the forms of space are not approached from outside, by attempting to apply ready made co-ordinate systems to them, but by entering into them and learning to understand the phenomena through their own mutual relationships. Through the fact that "the new geometry teaches us to live in the forms ... we are stimulated to study that mood of soul which, when developed further, leads us to penetrate into the supersensible world".

Humanity will be led through the present phase of materialism towards a time when the light of the spirit will shine again. To be more exact, humanity must itself struggle actively towards this future state. One-sided atomistic thought forms will be supplemented by other concepts and man's way of thinking will be more spiritual. Those who will be able to work powerfully towards this end will be the ones whose thinking has remained free, those who have experienced the new conception of space in their thinking and feeling have been able to realize it in their willing.

Bothmer regarded his work as a beginning. We must tend and cultivate this work and the many seeds that are to be found in it, that a gymnastics based on a living, spiritual conception of Man, together with a science which accords with the spiritual nature of the World, may be brought to the children in our schools.

Notes and References

1. George Adams and Olive Whicher: "The Plant between "Sun and Earth", 1952. "The Living Plant and the Science of Physical and Ethereal Spaces", 1949. Goethean Science Foundation, Clent, Stourbridge, England.

2. Rudolf Steiner: Lectures in The Hague, 8-10 April, 1922. Published in "Oesterreichische Blätter für freies Geistesleben". 6. Jahrgang, Vienna 1929.

3. G. Adams Kaufmann: "Von dem Aetherischen Raume". Natura, Medizinische Sektion am Goetheanum, 1933 (6. Jahrgang, Heft 5/6). English edition: "Physical and Ethereal Spaces", Anthroposophy,
London and New York, Volume 8, Nos. 3/4.

4. Rudolf Steiner: "Der Mensch - eine Hieroglyphe des Weltenalls", Lecture 1, Dornach, 9. April 1920 (Mathematisch-Astronomische Blatter, Heft 2, Dornach 1940.)

(See also: - G. Adams Kaufmann: "Strahlende Weltgestaltung", Mathematische-Astronomische Sektion am Goetheanum, Dornach, 1934. L. Locher-Ernst: "Projektive Geometrie", Orell-Fussli Verlag, Zurich 1940; "Zur mathematischen Erfassung des Gegenraumes", Math.-Astronomische Blätter, Heft 3, Dornach 1941. And: - Louis Locher-Ernst: Raum und Gegenraum. Mathematisch-Astronomische Sektion am Goetheanum, Dornach 1957.)

Gymnastic Education related to the Child's Development

The Path of Gymnastic Education

Fritz von Bothmer

Introduction

Man determines Space

He stands upright and lifts his head freely - to the Heights.

He falls - into the Depths.

He stands firmly with both feet on the earth and spreads out his arms –
to the Widths.

He directs his vision and his step forward towards a goal; thus he measures
out the Length.

He feels the force of resistance - backward.

With his arms, he traces the encircling round; they are the rays (radii).
The form of his head is a picture of the encircling sphere.

Thus Man impresses his stamp upon Space.

Man's consciousness it is, which distinguishes between the dimensions,
giving them meaning and measure. His consciousness is the center,
it determines direction and it is woven into the encircling sphere.

A School of Movement which, through the manifold play of forces in human movement, leads the growing child to experience boundless Space, ever and again bringing it to life and determining it according to the picture of man, will allow Space itself to arise in consciousness as the greater Man within man. It will overcome the dead conception of the three dimensions, finding instead a whole world of moral forces speaking dynamically through them, - a world which has already penetrated the idiom of human speech. Movement itself provides the guiding lines for such a school; movement which the pupil can follow with his senses and his consciousness, to the forces of which he will give form and measure. Such is the meaning and intention of the sequence of exercises here described.

Someone actually practicing the exercises will have no great difficulty in experiencing the fullness of a living conception of space, for he will be lead directly to this by the very movements themselves; indeed, they ask to be expressed out of such deeper experiences of space. The child accepts these movements quite naturally, and with a quiet happiness, for he feels himself widened and uplifted by them. For the reader, however, it will not be easy merely from the written description to make correct pictures of the movements without losing his way, unless he is able to be very active inwardly in following the dynamic sequences of movement.

Each one of the exercises described is complete in itself; each is a whole, a movement-picture into which the child can grow. Many details must be included here which will perhaps make the reader's task all the more difficult, for he will be trying to follow the movements pictorially. But these details will often be a very important help to anyone actually taking up this work in gymnastic education.

Physiological terms have been avoided. This is in keeping with the nature of a school of gymnastic movement, the first aim of which is to place the human being truly into the great organism of space and its prevailing forces. Upon this foundation he will then rightly learn to know the physiological forces of his own body.

The sequence of exercises covers a period of twelve school years, embracing the whole of gymnastic education. The exercises arose one after the other in the course of working with children between the ages of nine to eighteen years, boys and girls together. They changed their form often enough, before each single exercise and then the whole sequence really emerged. While writing, the author looks back to the years from 1922 to 1938 in the Waldorf School, Stuttgart, when this work in educational gymnastics came into being and grew. It was based simply upon the confidence given to the author by Dr. Rudolf Steiner, the educational director of the Waldorf School, who appointed him as teacher of gymnastics, giving him full scope and freedom. When Rudolf Steiner died in 1925, this school of gymnastics was still in its infancy, but he had given it his approval.

The gymnastics exercises were practiced in large mixed classes, together with work on the apparatus and with athletics and games. By 1926, the whole sequence of exercises was already there in broad outline, and its development was shown in public performances from year to year. The author is deeply indebted to Rudolf Steiner and the teachers and scholars of the Waldorf School, who so warmly supported him in his effort to establish this new approach to gymnastics.

The essence of this school is to use the play of forces at work in human movement in such a way as to evoke the ideal picture of greater Man living in infinite space, according to which the finite and limited human body will adapt itself and grow. The opposing force of gravity, or weight, will then be encountered, whose ultimate expression would be the fall, which, if it does not paralyze, awakens and stimulates man's strength of will.

Every heavy body, even the human body, is subject to the tendency to fall; this is revealed in every movement. Our movements either follow the tendency towards falling, either they succumb sooner or later to the force of gravity, or they counteract it. This involves the use of the limbs, directed by the will. This will may express itself merely as animal instinct; but man's will is capable at every degree of enhancement, culminating in the conscious resolve.

Even standing quietly upright, man is all the time overcoming with his will the tendency to give in to the force of gravity and to fall. When he is tired or unconscious he does fall. His power to remain erect ceases when the forces either of his will or of his consciousness become ineffective.

In the limit, the fall leads to an absence of gymnastic movement, to mere prostration. When this has happened, man has exchanged the vertical for the horizontal.

In jumping, he lifts his weight, releasing it momentarily from the earth. The more he is able to do this, the more forcibly must he react to gravity as he returns to the ground.

Gymnastics is man's consciously sustained endeavor to counteract the process of falling, in the most diverse conditions, where states of stability and balance are constantly changing. This is a schooling of the greatest educational value.

Falling takes place to begin with according to a physical law and the movement which comes about as a result of it, will take its course mechanically. These physical, mechanical laws are involved in all human movement; they are at work in the skeletal and muscular system. In mastering these laws, the child develops strength and agility, and gymnastics is indeed a training of the body.

Every free gymnastic movement takes place in space and time. Height, depth, width, breadth, length, forward, backward - these are not just dead concepts, but may be experienced as directing forces, uniting man with infinite space. The three dimensions - up and down, from side to side, forward and backward - are axes of space, but they are also axes of movement. They are built into man's body, - even into his organs of balance. Movement, in relating itself to these dimensions, brings them to living manifestation and even creates them. Such forms, and also the curves made by movement, are geometrical in character. To perceive and form them consciously demands an activity of thinking whereby one is fully aware of one's own movements and able to picture them in space.

But movement also has duration in time. I lift my arm sideways and upward and lower it again to the other side. The movement may give rise to a rhythm in time, - the rhythm of the circle - which will either submit to the force of gravity, when at last the swing comes to an end; or it may be caught up and continued, accelerated or changed. It might also be stopped abruptly. Thus, the rhythm may take its natural course and finally die away, or it may be developed and formed to something more. Rhythm comes about in the interplay of forces; it is the breathing of a movement, and it can be perceived through the feeling life of the pupil's rhythmic system.

The pupil should experience the power of the fall as an enduring force foreign to himself, over which he must always have mastery when he is moving. He must learn persistently to prevail over this force through constantly renewed resolves to movement. As a young child he will feel, and then later he will understand, how to give measure and direction to the movements and to keep his balance within them. The true meaning of the play of force in human movement will then dawn on him and he will hear the speech of that greater man within him. Through his thinking, feeling and willing, the instinct for movement will be lifted out of the animal sphere into the ethical and moral.

The truth, strength and beauty of a movement will testify to its rightness; the single movements in an exercise and the exercises in sequence follow one another out of their own objective inner necessity. The movement-pictures arrange themselves step by step into a world-picture. Thus the gymnastic exercises are a way of growth and development through human movement, and this is true education.

The child before us in class has at his disposal naturally given forces whereby he grows, stands upright, moves and becomes formed. The grown-up, however, must have made these forces his very own; he must have given them the stamp of his awakened consciousness, and therefore he stands there as an "I" in earthly space.

The time of puberty is the most outstanding period of development during the school years, and it presents the educator with the most arduous of his tasks. At this time, the young human being begins to be more independent in his thinking, feeling and willing. He is leaving the land of childhood, in which as a healthy child lighthearted and lightfooted, he was scarcely conscious of his body. Now, during the years of adolescence it may happen that he will sink down into the heaviness of his physical body, - with all the problems that this entails, and be given over to the material, mechanical aspect, unless qualities and capacities, above all of an artistic nature, are called forth within him. In the sequence of gymnastic exercises, this threshold of development is marked by the "Fall and its overcoming", around which the gymnastic work is centered in the 13th and 14th years. This appears in the exercises in two main forms, which will be variously modified. It is the first exercise which represents the decisive step into the third dimension, - into space; earlier exercises did not contain a definite step forward, but their movements remained more or less in planes and surfaces.

Three-dimensional space having at last been reached, the significant theme in the exercises will be the attaining of an individually chosen goal. In this the will is addressed most strongly of all; it is called forth in the striving to attain a goal, given a new task to fulfill. From the age of 15 and 16 onward, movement which has a conscious aim or goal is of most essential value. This also finds expression in exercises involving stepping and walking.

Thus a greater man emerges; a being who comes from Time and lives in Space. He rises above the mere technique of movement, and a life-force filled with purposes and meaning comes to him from Space itself.

Just as man bears neither male nor female distinguishing features other than in his physical body, so the exercises in the first group are not characteristically adapted to either sex. These earlier exercises are like a common root-stock from which the later ones - the "Fall into the Inclined plane" and the "Vertical fall" or "Fall into the point" - develop. The latter, the "Fall into the point", is an exercise containing great possibilities in movement, full of the opportunity to overcome difficulties. The former, which could also be called "Fall into Space", has two variations, each with equal richness of movement, one stressing more the quality of will, the other rhythm. Carried out by alternating groups of children, some doing one form and some the other, the exercise is a whole, in time and space. The "Fall and its overcoming" lends itself especially well to this, but many of the other exercises can be done in parts and in groups; in this way the particular note struck by a single exercise becomes the more impressive and its meaning in the whole sequence the more evident.

The social character of the exercises too is thus affirmed, and this may be enhanced to a high degree of dramatic tension. The roundelay at the end of this essay gives some impression of what is here meant*; it is a summing up of the various stages throughout the years.

That there is an inner necessity determining the way the movements follow one another in each single exercise and in the sequence as a whole, becomes clearer and clearer as we proceed. It arises simple from a deep contemplation of movement itself. This inner law and truth shows itself to be the guiding thread, rooted in the spiritual nature of man, which can, through the gymnastic movement, unite him once more with the forces of his spiritual origin.

---

* Omitted in the translation; it is a long verse intended as accompaniment to four exercises done in a group. (Pages 89-91 in the German.)

The Time before Puberty

First Roundelay (Ninth Year)

We come, we come from far and wide,
A-running and a-springing,
Gallop, gallop and trot, trot, trot
Gallop, gallop and trot, trot, trot
A-running and a-springing.

There stands for us a house built here,
Sound, as we shall tell;
Come now, let us look at it,
It will please us well.

Span wide the ring,
Each firm as a nail;
No-one among us
The others will fail.

Pillars are towering tall,
Windows so wide.
Come within, big and small,
Two side by side.

Open the windows out
Wide o'er the land

Heaven high, winging wide,
Firmly we stand.

Windows close!
Repose!

Shut and open,
Open and shut;
Wider open,
Once more shut.
See, you and I.

You and I, I and you
Seek one another, find one another,
Seek one another, find one another.
You and I, I and you.
See! See!

We've built a house and built it well
On rock and not on sand.
Pillars so high,
Windows so wide,
So shall it stand.
Tun-ta-ra-la-tum-ta-ra-la...

Plate 3

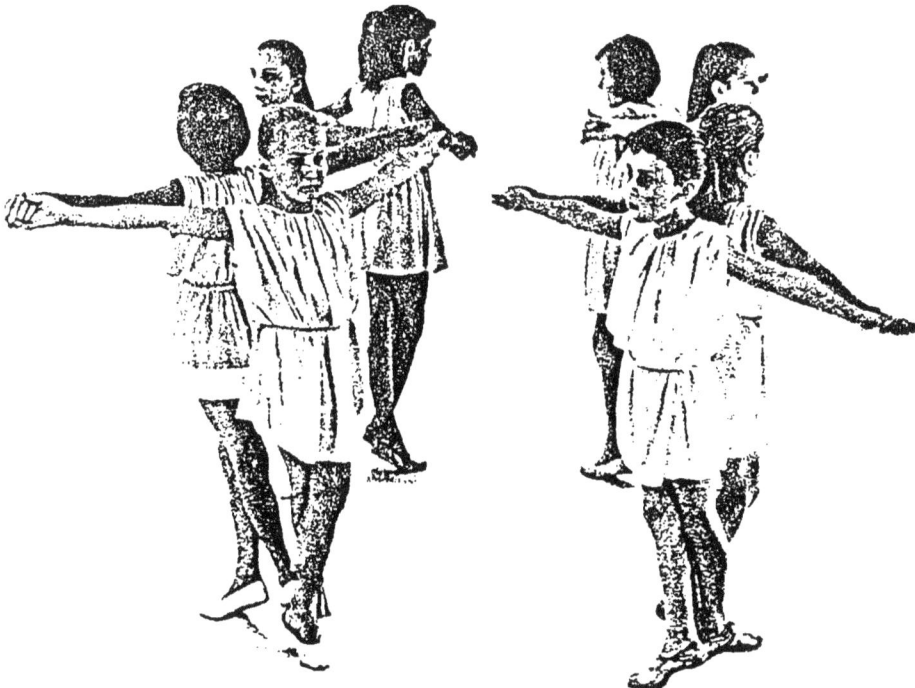

The children stand, boys and girls, in a circle. They take hands in pairs and then turn so that the pairs stand behind one another. The teacher then begins to speak the roundelay, emphasizing its rhythm, and the children, in pairs to begin with, start to move round the circle, running and jumping. At the end of the first verse they again form one large circle and come to a standstill at the end of the second verse. Stamping the rhythm of the verse as they step, the children span the circle as wide as possible and, coming to a halt, they let go hands.

The "pillars" appear as they jump to their toes with arms raised high above their heads: the "windows" as they spring feet apart and spread their arms wide. Then, with a jump, feet come together again and the children, two by two, face one another and hold hands.

Now each pair slips beneath the two arms which are nearest the outside of the circle; they turn on their toes and pass underneath, back to back. Coming through, they stand back to back on tiptoe, still holding hands, with arms extended wide apart and legs crossed. Then follows "Heaven High", when arms are raised high and lowered again sideways to "Winging wide". In the strongly spanned tension of this last movement, legs, which are still crossed, stand firmly on the ground.

The children then face one another again in pairs and turning back again on toes, they pass beneath the same two uplifted arms. This is repeated, now turning under the other two arms. "Wider open" is depicted when, while holding hands all the time, with upstretched arms, one of the two children remains standing and allows the other to move right round him, turning as he does so, until at last they face one another again. This movement is repeated alternately by each child in the pair, with the words "You and I", so that they move on a kind of figure-of-eight to each two lines. After the last "I and you", all the children turn towards the center of the circle and clap their hands at "See! See!".

The children then step and clap the beat, converging towards the center of the circle and moving out again, and then they repeat the "Heaven high" and "Winging wide" movements. Then, with a jump, they bring feet together again, make a half turn and follow one another round the circle with outspread arms to the rhythm of "Turn-ta-ra-la".

The circle then changes to an inward moving spiral, until the movement becomes congested towards the center. The children then turn, hold hands, and quickly open the spiral out again to a circle.[*]

---

[*] In this Roundelay Bothmer often started with the children standing in pairs in a corner of the hall, so that the circle was gradually formed as they ran; then after the spiral he would also end, not in a circle, but by letting the children disperse into the widths, from whence they came.

Second Roundelay (Ninth Year)

I stand,
I walk ...
I run o'er the ground ...
I leap, I leap
And halt without sound.

I leap on the wall,
And swing to the tower,

To ring the bell, to ring the bell ...
That strikes the hour.

Far and wide,
And wide and high,
And still wider ...
I stand.

Plate 4

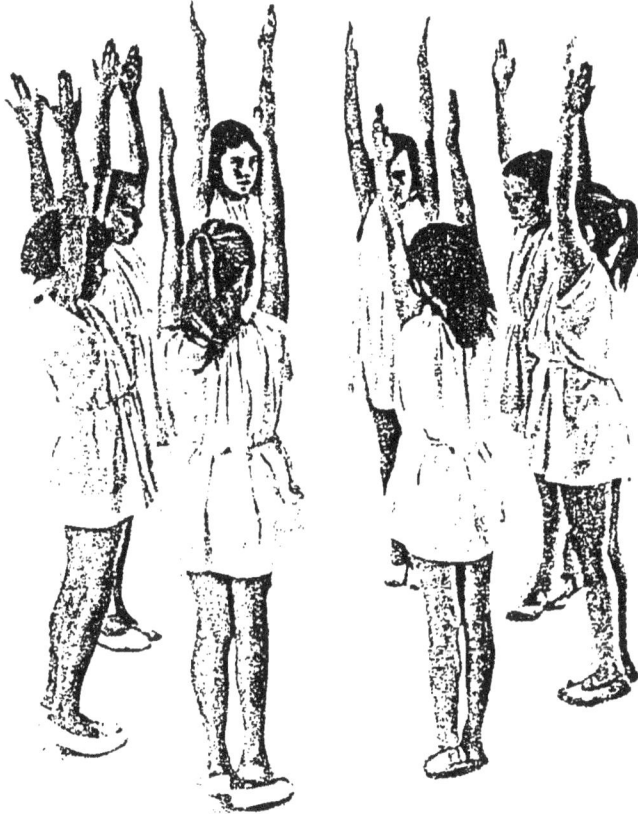

The children stand in a circle and then turn so that they are in single file behind one another. The teacher speaks the roundelay with a strong rhythm.

The children stand upright, heels together, firmly on the ground; then they walk, upright but easily, one behind the other; then they run, and while running, they hold themselves naturally.

The leaps, strong and high, go with the rhythm of the spoken word ($\cup$ -, $\cup$ -)

Gradually, the running comes to a standstill and the children turn towards the center of the circle. Then they jump to feet apart and open their arms wide. The "wall" stands there, strong and wide!

The children then let their arms fall and swing down across one another to the front, like a swing of the pendulum; the returning swing is carried right up to height, both arms swinging sideways and up, bringing the whole body with them. The "lower" stands, tall and slim!

The ringing of the bell is a rhythmical swinging movement, led by the arms* as though they were pulling the rope and reaching from height to depth and back. The ringing ends with a vigorous jump, in which the body reaches up as high as possible. The jump should be easy and springy and the arms accompany it by making a wide circle, coming right down sideways and then swinging up again in front to the horizontal, bringing the body up again after the jump. The arms then show the sound of the bells going out ...

"Far and wide, wide and high,
And still wider... *

The children slowly lower their arms again and stand quietly and firmly on both feet once more.

These roundelays are gymnastic exercises for the small children; they can be repeated again and again. Single movements may be practiced separately - also the running and jumping - but these should then always be reintroduced into the roundelay.

It is much better to demonstrate movements, rather than to attempt to explain them; and the rhythm of the movement is of no less importance than the form.

*

Little exercises such as the following may well be introduced between the roundelays, or especially at the beginning of the lesson:

"Stand, wide and strong, on your two feet and raise your right fore-finger as high as you can! Now keep your feet firmly on the ground and with your finger show me your left toe. 'There is my left toe'. Now stand up again and raise your left fore-finger high and show me your right toe..." Or: "hold hands in a circle; with your right toe, show me your left toe... and now your left knee. 'That is my left toe and, - that is my left knee'. Point on point and point on stump!" Or:

"Lay your left hand flat on your back, as high as you can; now try to make your right hand grasp the left one. Whoever can hold hands firmly, may dance round in a circle..." This may be done with alternating hands.

*

---

* From height, forward to depth
** With the words, "Far and wide" arms are raised sideways, with "and" twice forward, the third time to widths again, but palms turned upward. This leads the arms upward to height, "and still wider" beyond height they "grow to widths", - a movement which is practiced more consciously later on. (See page 16).

Third Roundelay

(10th, 12th Year)

Go round the circle,
Step by step,
Tread by tread,
Hour after long hour
Together we tread.

My road goes this way,
Your road goes that way;
That way goes your road,
This way goes my road.

Give me your two hands,
Turn round and round...

Now it's all over,
Hope we're still sound!

Go round the circle,
Step by step,
Tread by tread,
Hour after long hour
Together we tread.

Tschin-tschin, tschin, tschin, tschin
Tschin, tschin, tschin, etc.
Rum-rum, bum, bum, bum etc.

Plate 5

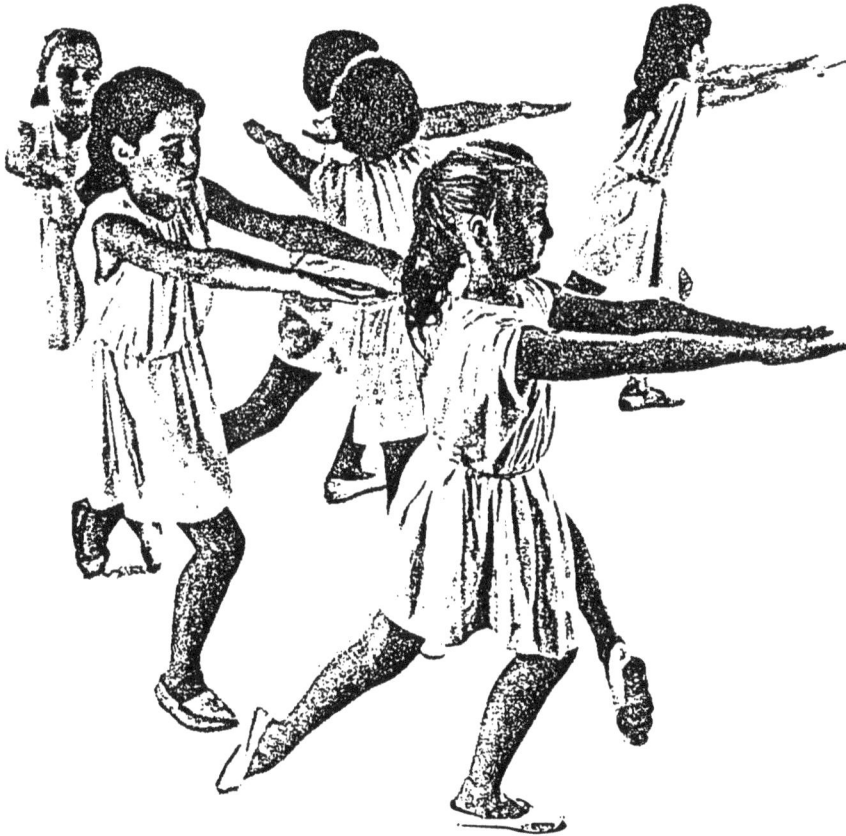

The children stand in two concentric circles, boys in one, girls in the other. They march round behind one another keeping step to the rhythm, boys one way, girls the other, and beating time with their hands on imaginary drums and cymbals. Then each child takes a falling step forward (a lunge), at the same time bringing one or both arms forward, to point in the direction in which he is going. With a quick turn on their toes, they then do the same in the opposite direction. This is repeated, and then the children jump forward again on to both feet, facing in the direction in which they began.

27

Then boys and girls in pairs take one another by both hands and with feet near together, leaning back with outstretched arms, they spin round quickly on their toes, like a top. When the spinning slows down and stops, the pairs shake hands and each child turns again in his original direction. The movement belonging to the first verse is then repeated.

Before the first and after the last verse, the teacher can make the children march found, stamping the rhythm of the rhyme and imitating the movements of beating drums and cymbals.

*

The roundelays contain spatial concepts in picture form. Height, depth, width, breadth - all are woven into them. "Pillars so high", "Windows so wide", "Leap on the wall", "Swing to the tower", "Ringing the bells", - all these form the basis for gymnastic movement and help the child to feel how he is set into space.

The forward direction, involved as it is in the reaching of a consciously chosen aim or goal, comes in the more formal gymnastic movement only later on, at the age of fourteen and fifteen years; this corresponds to the child's development in consciousness. In the roundelay, the idea of direction towards a goal appears in picture form,

"My road goes this way;
your road goes that way".

The young child does of course already have this experience in the natural way, but it is not yet emphasized and brought to full consciousness in a gymnastic exercise. In the upper school, however, when thinking takes hold of the will, the conscious setting of an aim or goal and its attainment becomes a central theme in the gymnastic lessons.

The roundelays also take into account the stage of physical and psychological development reached by the child. The two roundelays:

"We come, we come from far and wide," and "I stand, I walk..." are suited to children from about the ninth to the eleventh year. The last: "Go round the circle" belongs to the tenth and twelfth years. After this the child will have outgrown the roundelays; from the point of view of gymnastics, he will stand on his own feet. The change to the next stage should, however, be made gradually.

It is quite conceivable that gymnastic exercises in the form of roundelays and accompanied by the spoken word might also be practiced in the upper school; it would be pure gymnastics. In the lower school, the roundelays are a natural element in which the young children find community together, the fantasy pictures in them forming the ground out of which more formal gymnastic movements can grow. Later on, in the higher classes, it is conscious and intensive gymnastic striving which brings the individual to realize, in rhythmic and dramatic group forms, the true value of his own effort. This can then lead to the creating of a higher form of comradeship and community. A roundelay such as this final one might well be accompanied by music instead of the spoken word.

* * *

Play between Weight and Lightness

Just as movements may be taken from the roundelays and developed into exercises, so these first exercises give rise to further ones, leading over directly to the next epoch of child development. While at first our aim was to help the child to find his way happily and truly into the world of space, now a new element enters in. It may be described as the "Play between Weight and Lightness".

Man, standing upright, is poised between the downward pull of gravity and the working of another force. This force draws upward, away from the earth; it is the very antithesis of gravity and may therefore be called "levity".

As the child approaches puberty, he begins to feel this contrast in himself, and this is taken up by the gymnastic method and gives the exercises their content. The interplay of these two great and divergent forces is a dynamic one. It may result in catastrophe, - the fall; or it may mean the turning of the scales, - change and metamorphosis. The roundelay having made three-dimensional space real for the child, the exercises which follow establish an easy, lively relationship between heights and depths and then lead him further in his experience of the way space is formed and articulated.

Example:

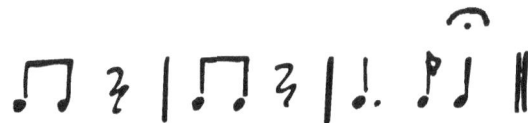

Jump astride, at the same time lifting the arms sideways to the horizontal, and them jump lightly back again. Repeat. Repeat a third time, but bring the arms right up to the vertical; a short jump brings feet together and the arms are then lowered again to the standing position.

Example:

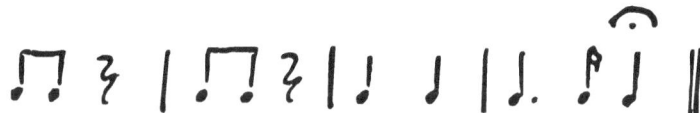

The same movement as above. After the third jump, both arms swing right down forward and between the legs and then, as they swing up again to the vertical, the whole body springs up with a jump which brings the feet together; return to standing position.

These two simple but strong rhythms can be practiced alternately or together; for example, one by the girls and the other by the boys at the same time, keeping to the rhythm given by the teacher.

A further example of the play between "weight" and "lightness", the widths, the heights and the depths.

Example:

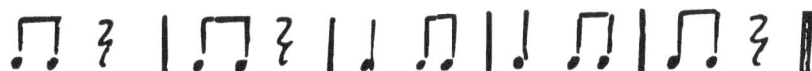

Two light jumps, feet astride with arms lifted sideways to width, and back again to the balanced standing position. (Weight). then a third similar jump to width and from there a simple hopping movement on toes, either keeping the legs together or alternately setting one foot before the other. (Lightness).

Plate 6

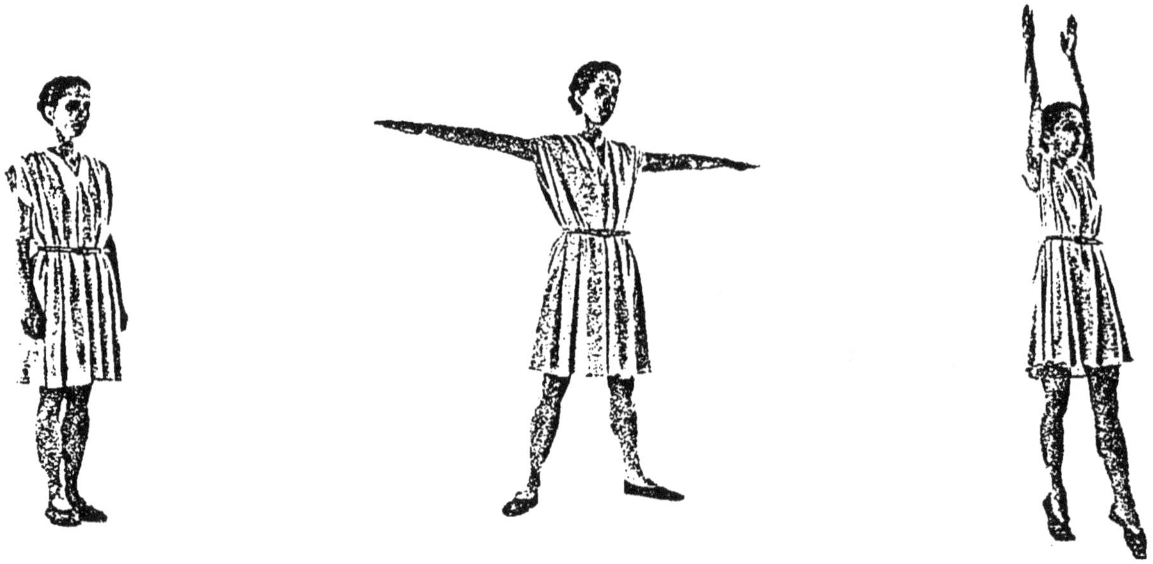

The teacher may give the rhythm of the exercise by speaking:

"Hea–vy,
Hea–vy,
Heavy – light, light
Heavy – light, light
Hea–vy"

The rhythm might also be varied to a five-fold one, by inserting extra steps in the light beats. A quarter turn might be made at the moment of jump into weight and forward skipping steps in the jumps in lightness; for example, boys and girls might do alternate variations.

Another example:

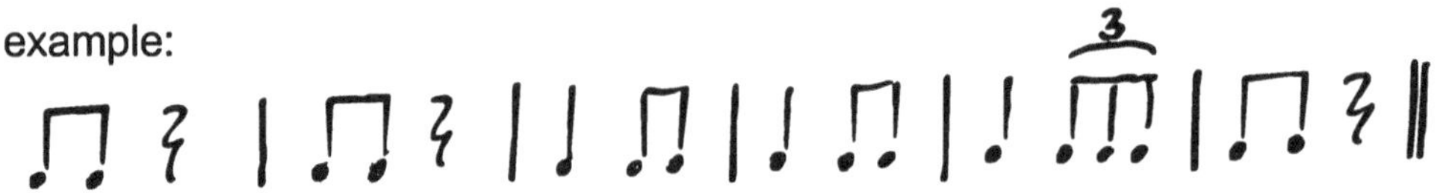

The exercise may also be enhanced if, during the jump into weight, the arms, long and relaxed, are lifted to the horizontal, while with the light hopping movements, they swing upward to height. The spoken rhythm would then be:

"Wi-den
Wi-den,
Wide – high, high
Wide – high, high
Wi-den"

The experience of width is especially gained through the participation of the arms, and the movement flows freely with the unrestricted stream of the breath. In this, as indeed, in all the exercises, it is the upper part of the body which takes the lead in the movement.

30

Attention should always be given to foot movements. The feet are by nature often very skillful, even though physically they are the parts of the body most remote from consciousness. The wonderful build of the human foot is peculiar to man, and it accords with the nature of the feet that they should be developed into sensitive organs of touch. They often have to start off a movement, and consciousness should be directed down to them, so that the steps they take may have meaning and purpose. It is by virtue of the finely articulated joints, one upon the other, of feet and legs, that these limbs are able to play their part in counteracting and overcoming gravity. All exercises, therefore, which call upon the activity of the feet are useful in awakening the capacities of the whole human being.

Equally valuable for this awakening process is the effort to bring to consciousness the spatial forms that arise during movement. It is good for the pupil to learn to follow quite exactly what forms come about, either on the floor or in space, when he moves; and the simple exercises just described afford excellent opportunity to make a beginning in this. From time to time he should watch for himself how his feet are moving on the floor or his hands around him in space. The grown-up may do well to draw such forms on paper, as seen for example from above, in front or from the side. The exercises should however have first been mastered gigantically.

Each exercise may be understood and practiced from three aspects; the forming of space, the rhythm and the sheer dynamic force. Of these three, to be conscious of the form requires a certain degree of mental awareness and geometrical understanding, while over-emphasis upon physical force debases gymnastic movement and stresses the animal element in it.

Rhythm belongs to the very nature of movement, especially to the movements of a child. It establishes a harmony between above and below, between the cool, formative process of thinking and the chaotic, fiery impulses of will. Rhythm is a healing force, belonging to the middle system in man, recreated ever and again in the flow of breathing, and the pulse of the blood.

Gymnastic rhythms should be objective, that is to say, they should arise out of the movement itself and not be superimposed upon it. It would not be right to make up a rhythm, or borrow one from some piece of music, for example, and then try to fit it to a movement. Every good gymnastic movement will have its own rhythm, and once this is established, it is of course possible to create the accompanying words or music.

Plate 7

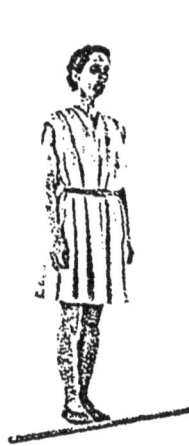
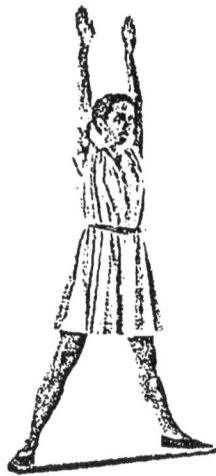
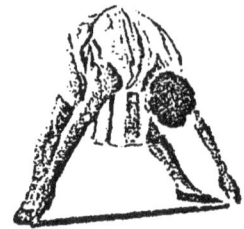

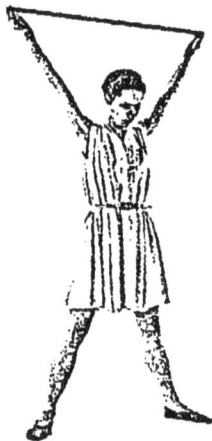
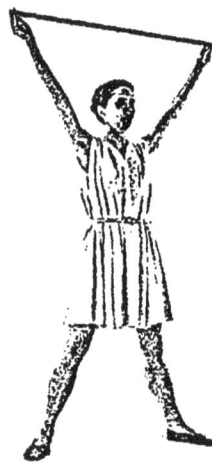
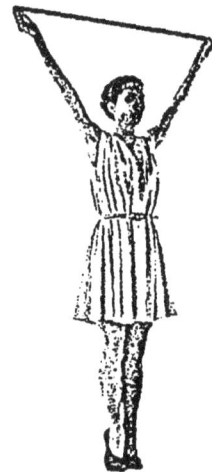

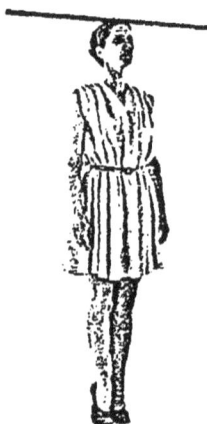
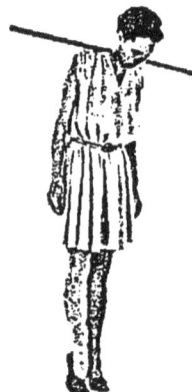
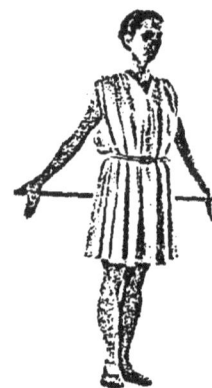

Triangle with Rod

Eleven to twelve year-olds may be led on from the preliminary exercises to the actual gymnastic exercises with the help of something taken from their other school work, namely, the triangle, which can inspire gymnastic movement from many aspects. Both in the play of forces and in the forming of space which it involves, this exercise is many-sided, yet easy to understand.

Teacher and children each take a wooden or copper rod in both hands! They lay them on the floor at their feet.*

> "The rod lies there. I stand.
> Below - above.
> Depths - heights.
> Horizontal - vertical.

"I stand firmly, feet as wide apart as the length of rod lying before me, arms raised upward. The vertical, the height, is thus brought nearer to the horizontal, the width. The height is built as triangle upon the horizontal base line given by the rod, the arms pointing upward to the apex.

"Height swings down to depth; it swings right through, and coming back, the arms separate and hands grasp the base line, the rod, at either end, carrying it upward to height. Two triangles appear momentarily, which are the reflection of one another, but as the upward movement culminates with the raising of the head to vertical, the feet come together with a jump on to the toes. The apex of the triangle is now below; the base line, width, is above.

"The triangle is standing on its apex."

"Now the base line, the rod, is carried down behind the head towards depth, to begin with as far as the middle of the back. Here a small central triangle is created. I stand firmly on the ground again.

"From the place behind the back, the base line springs up again,** passing over the head and down to depth, returning to its starting place."

> "There lies the rod once more."
> "I stand."

While the rod is moving down behind the back, it may pause for a moment and balance horizontally, first on the head and then on the shoulders, during which time the triangle still remains poised on its apex. Each time the rod is made to balance, arms are lowered to the sides.

A further enhancement of this exercise would be to bring the base line of the inverted triangle right down behind the back to the apex below, and then up again, just as before it was the apex which swung down forwards to the base line below.

The static triangle form is thus brought into movement, and in moving, it causes the body constantly to adjust itself to the changes of position it assumes; it creates rhythm; and it

---

* Bothmer worked with wooden rods and on one occasion he said they should be made of ash.
** The grip may be altered with both hands at once and then the rod is brought round to the front with one hand to be held by both hands as the arms - parallel - hang down.

brings to consciousness the manifold possibilities of the play of forms and forces in space. All this brings a feeling of harmony to the body.

Square with Rod

The square, practiced gymnastically, belongs naturally to the horizontal. The pupil assumes the position of a mid-point or a vertical axis in the center and builds the square around himself, one side after another, holding the rod shoulder-high and grasping it firmly at the ends. The rod forms the sides of the square, while the arms are like radii. Care is taken to see that the sides are all even and at the same height, with four well-made corners at right-angles, keeping the radii firm and unbroken. Then the square is taken away again, side after side.

The square is more akin to man's bony system than is the triangle; unlike the latter, it has no innate dynamic force and therefore no gymnastic rhythm. Alone through its rhythm, the triangle will inspire a gymnastic exercise. (See Plate 8)

Plate 8

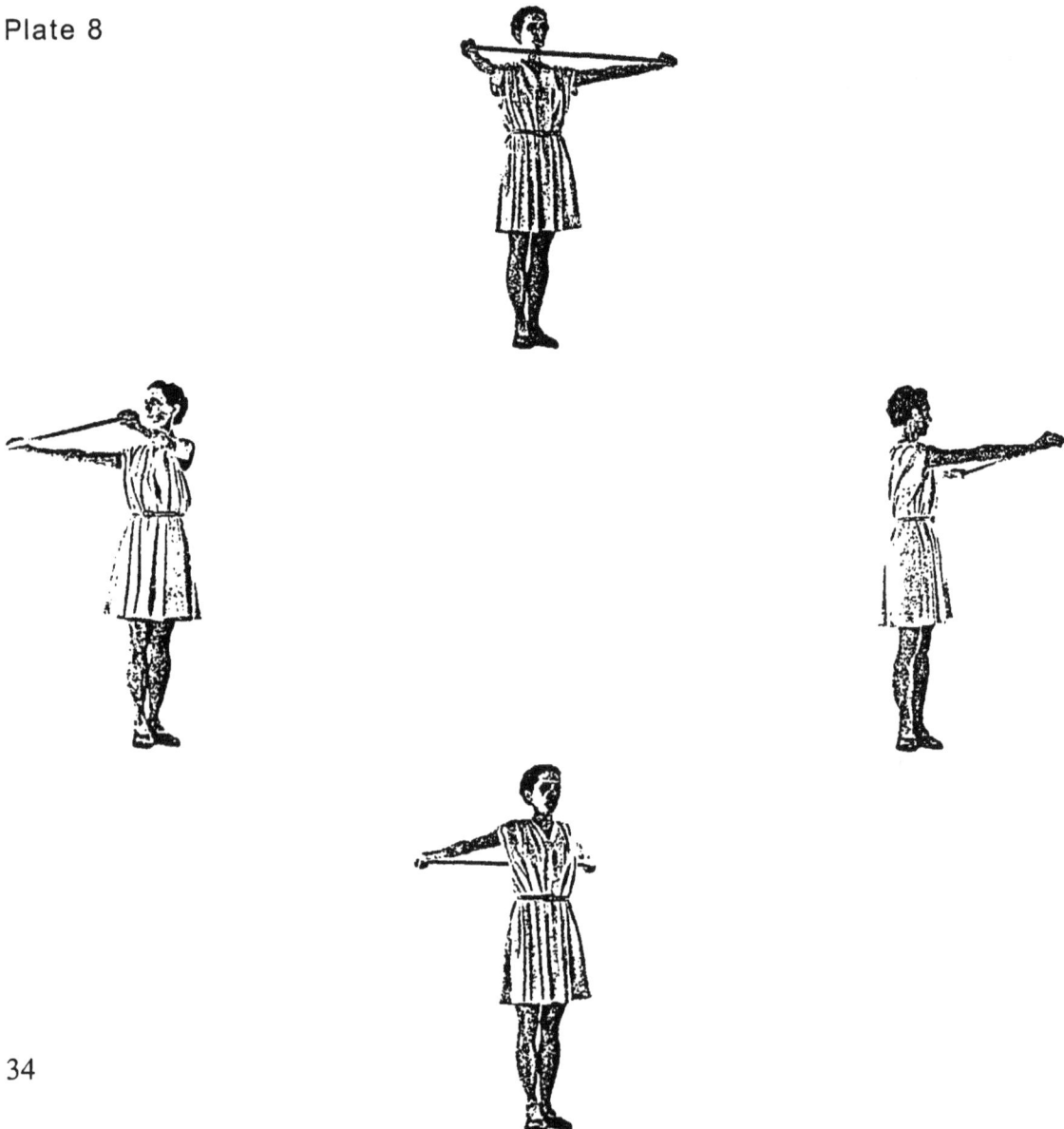

Triangle without Rod

In these gymnastic exercises it is the rod which gives the tangible measure. To do without the rod and simply hold the measure in consciousness, belongs to a later stage of development. In the triangle exercise done without a rod, the arms swing down, dividing as though to grasp the rod, and then simply take the measure of the distance between the feet and use it as base line for the triangle. The transformation of the triangle then follows in like manner as before. At the close, the pupil relaxes from the tension of the upside-down triangle and returns to the position "I stand".

From the moment when the apex swings down to the base line, the transformation of the triangle, done without a rod, is an experience of streaming forces.

Plate 9 – Triangle without rod

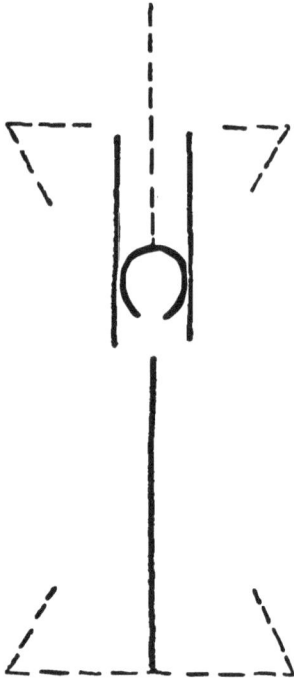

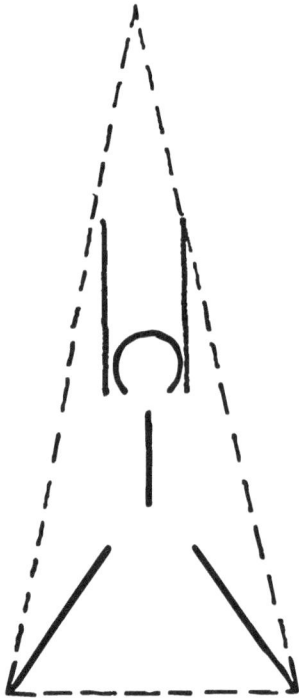

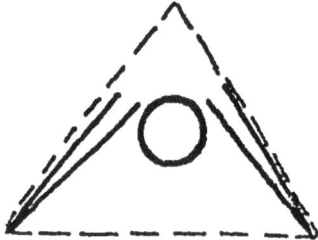

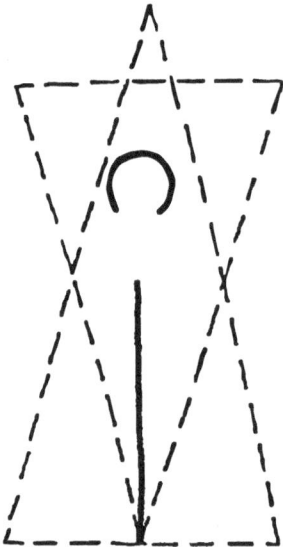

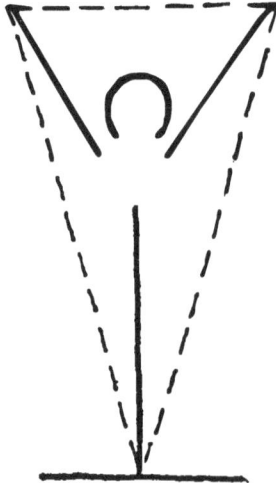

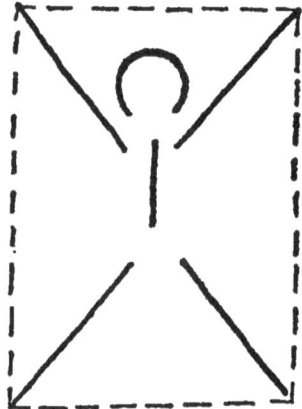

36

The Re-entrant Triangle

Quite a different movement picture arises in another exercise based on the triangle, if we imagine a force from above pressing downward, either steadily or suddenly, so that the apex of the triangle is pushed downward and inward towards the center. There is a strong muscular tension as the hands are clenched to fists; the forces which can otherwise stream freely in and out through the limbs, are thus dammed up in the muscles. This pent-up force strains for release, and when the arms are pushed powerfully downward and across one another, it shoots through the center of the triangle and out into the void, leaving the arms crossed rigidly in front of the body. It would then appear that the movement had reached a moment of frustration, until, seeking for space, the arms, still crossed, thrust upward over the head and back, meeting with a resistance against the nape of the neck. Tension is growing all the time. The re-entrant triangle (formed by the trunk and arms), its apex having been forced in by the pressure from above, seeks an apparent release, only to reach yet another moment of anti-climax. Now, however, a new force enters in, - the power of the up-right, vertical stature of man. It bears the body upward. The head is raised against the con-straint of the crossed arms, and as it reaches the vertical, the triangle, still compressed, springs to its apex (with a jump feet together on toes). Now the re-entrant triangle, still held in tension with arms and fists crossed in the nape of the neck, is standing on its apex, while the upward power of the vertical has raised the body to the position of utmost resistance. At this moment the tension is released, the arms open out wide and high as feet come to-gether on toes, to make the vertical triangle once more, before the arms, continuing on sideways and down, make a great circle to bring the movement to a close in the standing position.

"I stand".

The process of forming and transforming the re-entrant triangle is not as easy to follow as with the ordinary triangle. The pupil has to make the effort all the time to follow the apex of the triangle as it is pushed and pressed from place to place, not losing sight of it even in moments of greatest distortion. Only after a long sequence of thrusting movements does the apex of the triangle unexpectedly appear once more in the heights, and then the pupil should experience a great sense of liberation as the tension is released and the streaming power which has been pent up in the muscles is allowed to flow freely again.

Movement of this kind, where the force is dammed up in strong muscular tension, develops the muscles but easily hinders the free flow of the breathing. It may, however, be unwhole-some, if accompanied by deep breathing and if it is continually led over again rhythmically into free and flowing movement.

This is shown in a further development of this exercise which however, because of the de-mand it makes on consciousness and on the forces of balance and rhythm, belongs to a much older class.

Plate 10 – The re-entrant triangle

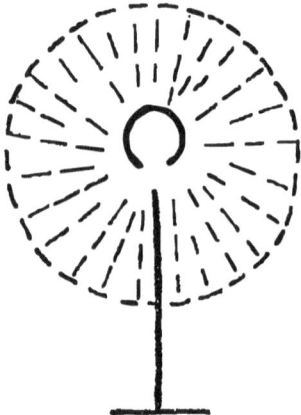

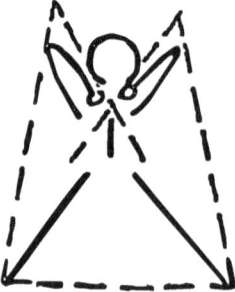

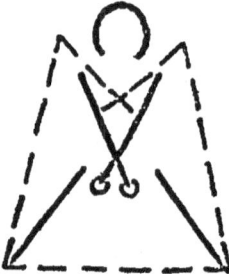

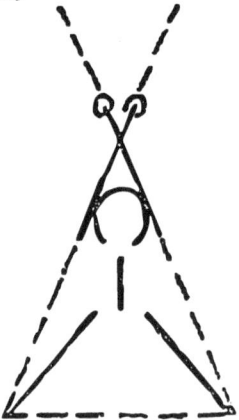

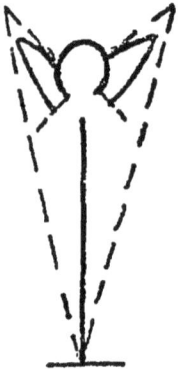

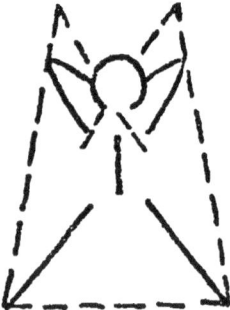

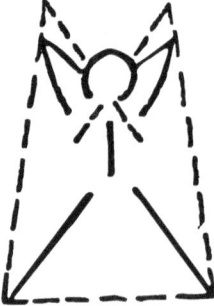

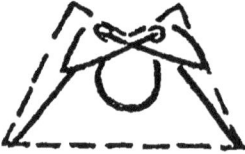

The rolling Rod

The following rod exercise, though not so outspokenly geometrical in character, requires a considerable feeling for space, a good sense of balance and agility.

The rod is held in front of the body, arms hanging down. It is then thrown upward with out-stretched arms and, remaining horizontal, is caught again on the backs of the hands and carried down, with a low bend of the body, to within a few inches of the floor. With a pow-erful forward and upward movement, the arms are raised until the rod begins to roll down them, over the bent head and the shoulders, and is caught again by both hands behind the back as the body straightens up. The arms, now hanging down and holding the rod behind the body, are then stretched out backward and raised, holding the ends of the rod and car-rying it upward again until, released by the hands, it rolls back down the arms to the neck. There it is again gripped by the hands from behind, lifted high above the head and brought down forwards in front of the body. The exercise takes place for the most part outside the pupil's field of vision.

Plate 11 – The rolling rod

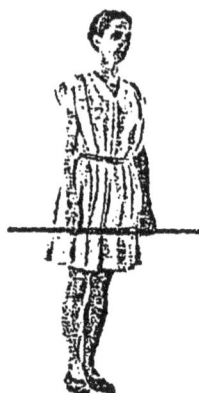

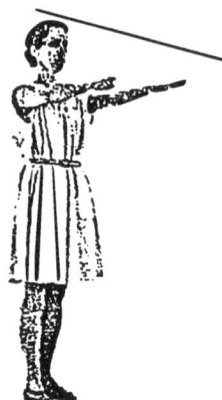

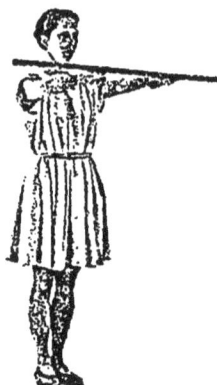

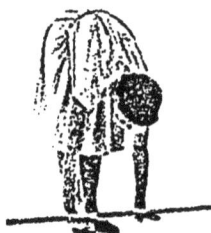

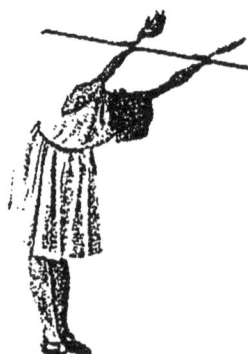

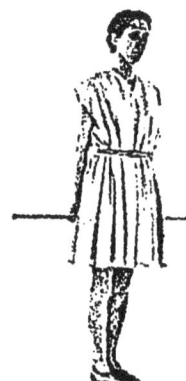

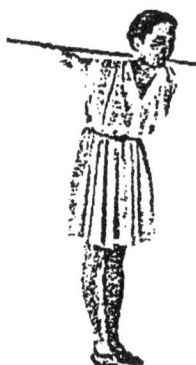

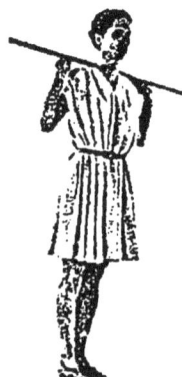

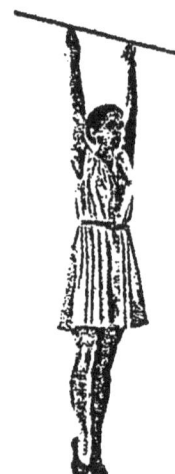

Sideways Circling

A great variety of space-forming and rhythmical gymnastic movements may be derived from the dynamic form of the circle. The following exercise belongs in its simpler form to the lower school, but it may be further developed to suit the middle and upper schools.

One arm, hanging loosely, is raised sideways (e.g. the right arm towards the left) and up over the highest point until it falls again on the other side and the movement comes to rest with a pendulum swing. The upward movement is brought about by human force, the fall by the force of gravity. Human force at first overcomes gravity and then gives way to it. A simple rhythm arises in this alternation of tension and relaxation which may be repeated, continued or accelerated. If the curve of the circle is widened as the arm falls from height to depth, a strong swing will be given to the circling movement which may be deliberately enhanced.

The pupil then allows himself to be taken hold of by the power of this swinging circling movement, rising and falling with it, turning as the movement requires, and is led into a kind of sideways stepping movement. Circling loops are developed from the circle, the swing of which can be enhanced by the pupil, while at the same time he is carried along both by the form and by the rhythm of the movement. Rhythm is fired by form and form by rhythm. A lively interplay arises between the pupil's own activity and the dynamic of the exercise as such. It can be followed either with complete abandonment to the whirling movement or with quiet attention to controlling the spatial form.

Higher demands may be made on the pupil's presence of mind and sense of space if the circling loops, having at first remained in one plane, are then carried into the third dimension. A turn is made between successive loops*, and though the body turns from side to side, the circling movement streams on uninterruptedly and the unity of the arm movements above and the stepping movement below is maintained. After practicing with one arm, the movements may e carried out with both arms swinging together, when the difficulty in keeping control of the form with its double loops is increased.

The simple rhythm remains unchanged throughout the variations:

The spontaneous run of the circling loops may be interrupted and formed again in the reverse direction by leading the last loop over the highest point of the circle and into a widely spanned inward moving spiral. The body is then held in balance by both feet and particularly by the outer one. The movement then returns, out of the depth of the spiral and, passing slowly over height, reverts to the circling rhythm, coming to a close again with the spiraling movement at the end of the run. The whole exercise is then like one great swing of a pendulum.

The spiral needs the skill and the consciousness of space which older pupils can bring to it, if it is not to degenerate into a merely mechanical movement.

---

* The turn is through 180 degrees, so that the loops still remain in one plane.

Plate 12 – Sideways circling

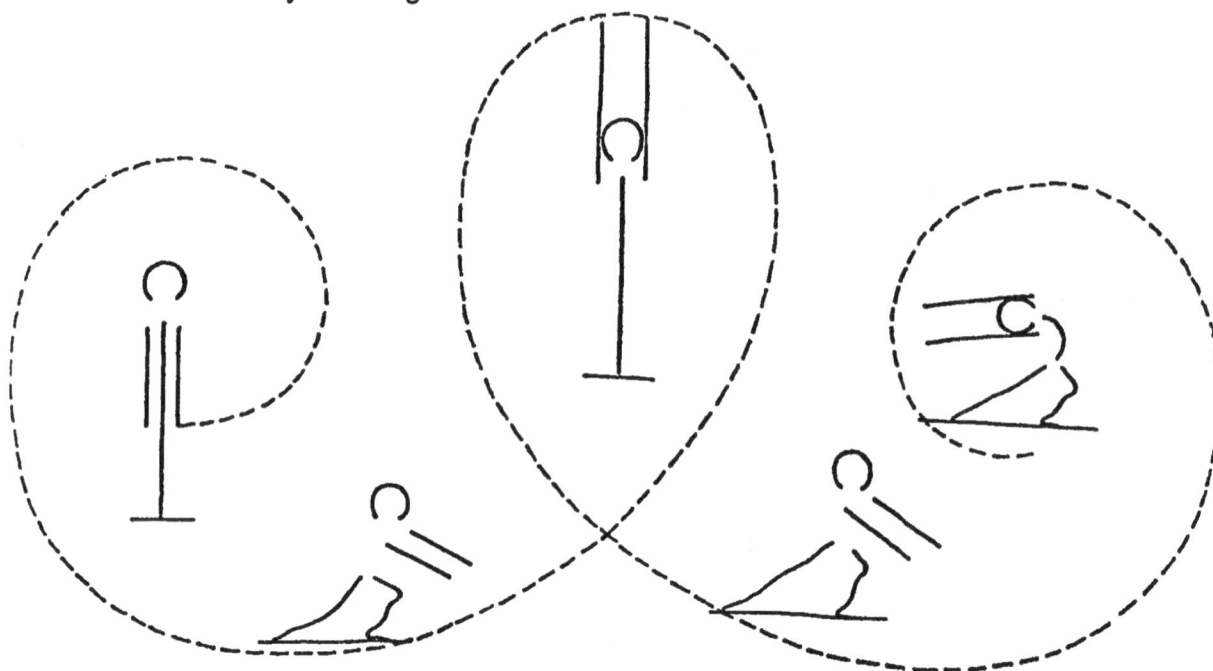

Jump into the Center

Upright man embodies and brings to expression the balanced interplay of upward and downward-streaming forces.

In jumping, man can to some extent attain the heights. In following the downward stream, his movement is arrested by the resistance of the earth.

The simplest way in which the interplay of these two forces comes to expression is in a light springy movement of the body up and down in the vertical line, - a movement in one dimension only. It can either be accentuated or allowed to die away, or it can be developed into something more. This springy movement, up and down on the toes, can be practiced at first with arms at rest and then with arms raised.*

If the movement develops upward, towards the heights, it may open out above into a great circle; the arms divide and move down on either side. The movement then swings through to the depths, where the two halves of the circle cross over, uncrossing when the arms reach the heights once more. This simple rhythmical exercise may be repeated, either by starting the springing movement again as soon as the arms reach the top of the circle, or by making a little jump and immediately opening the arms out again into the circle.

---

* Palms forward

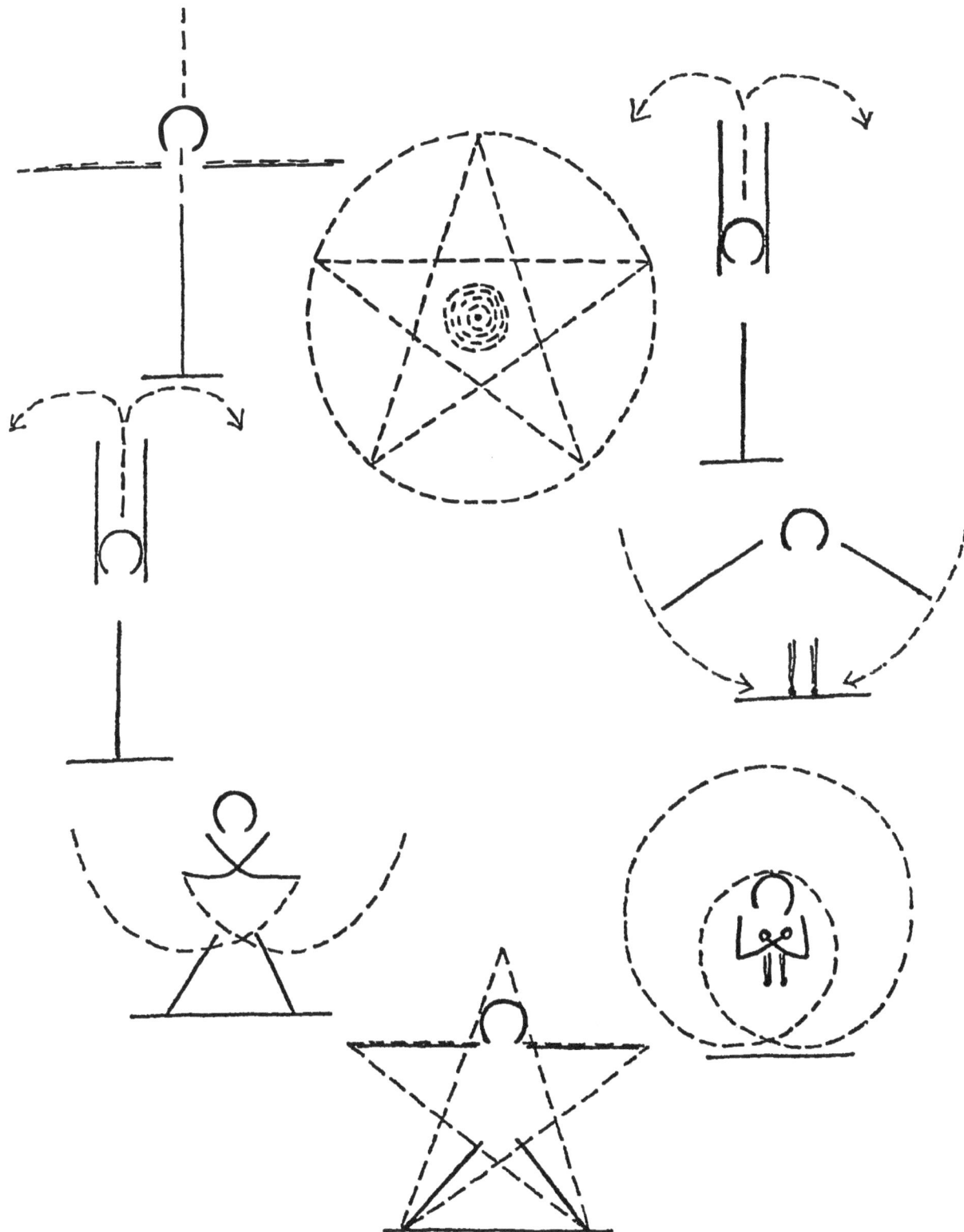

Plate 13 – Jump into the center

If the movement develops upward, towards the heights, it may open out above into a great circle; the arms divide and move down on either side. The movement then swings through to the depths, where the two halves of the circle cross over, uncrossing when the arms reach the heights once more. This simple rhythmical exercise may be repeated, either by starting the springing movement again as soon as the arms reach the top of the circle, or by making a little jump and immediately opening the arms out again into the circle.

The radii of the two halves of the circle cross when the lowest point has been passed, and during the return to height, this crossing-point goes through the mid-point of the great circle. Emphasis may be given to the mid-point, if the whole body is gathered up* for one moment into the center of the circle with a spring, which develops out of the swing of the encircling movement. As the two radii cross, the two halves of the circle, and "above" and "below", are drawn together to the center. This spring into the center of the circle is resolved and a state of balance regained when, after the rebound, the five-pointed star position is achieved; the limbs then radiate from the center and the movement comes to rest in the wide expanse. With a pendulum swing of the arms, the movement then returns to its origin in height.** This swing back to height may also be accompanied by a turn through 180 degrees.

Example of Music:***

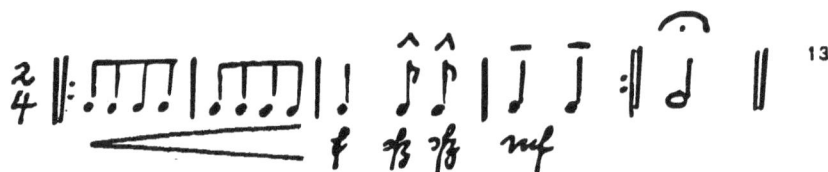

The unfolding of the heights into the wide circle, the momentary contraction of the circle into its center, and the subsequent movement, radiating from the center out into space, all of them strengthen the child's consciousness of space. There is a great opportunity for rhythm in the springing movement to height, the quiet circling movement which follows, the sudden jump which then comes completely to rest, and lastly in the pendulum swing. The exercise also addresses itself powerfully to the physical forces of the body.

The balance of forces in the five-pointed star, in which the widths play a great part, was derived from the spring into the center of the circle. This balance of forces can also arise if the pupil simply stands with feet wide apart and spreads his arms into the horizontalplane, taking this plane as the place from which the movement begins. The pendulum swing which then follows does not come to an end in height, but its rhythm carries it on towards a final state of balance in width. The swing to height grows into width; it is an enhancement of height beyond itself.*

   "Jump into breadth

---

* Hands made to fists.
** The exercise may be begun again from here; it can also be brought to an end here in the movement described in what follows as "grow to widths." This ending, as it was done by Bothmer, was also done as a single exercise. The movement "grow over height out into width" is like a quiet echo of the up and down springing movement and its subsequent development into the circle. The concentration inward, in the spring into the center is polar opposite to the movement reaching the widths in the second half of the exercise. For the first time in the sequence of exercises, the center arises as the crossing point of forces from two directions.
*** The springing movement at the beginning is done in this case in an 8/8 rhythm. The fewer the jumps, the more concentrated their crescendo. If they are altogether eliminated, the jump into the circle made by arm movements is immediate. The final note is "grow to widths."
* With breadth, the palms of the hands face downward, with width upward

Swing
To height,
Grow
To width".

Spanned into width, the pupil (and that means "width" itself), stands firmly on the ground...
"Finish" ... and then he releases the span into width and returns to the original position.

"I stand".

The Rhythm

The pupil may also descend out of the soaring heights and follow the other, opposing force which draws him earthward. Instead of letting the heights open out upward and become transformed into the circle, he swings down with long outstretched arms, forward and downward through the depths. The downward swing of the arms then follows through to width and brings him up again, with his arms resting in the balance of the horizontal. All at once the greatest width is confronted with the greatest contraction, and the movement, constrained for moment, is drawn forward so that the radii, right and left, cross in the horizontal plane. This crossing now becomes the center from which the movement swings upward into the heights and down again in a wide circle which encompasses the whole form. From its lowest point at the bottom of the circle, the movement returns to its origin in the heights.**

"Height to depth
to width -
Center
Ray out to circle
Depth to height".

Example of music:

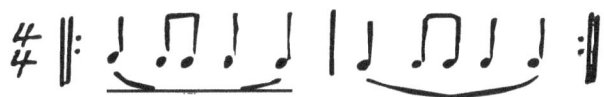

** The palms of the hands face forward or downward throughout the movement. Hands and arms are as one in the swinging movement. The independence of the hands comes in the next exercise. The feeling of opening out to height from the crossing point and the experience of rhythm are deepened, and the movement enriched, if a turn is made when the movement reaches its apex, so that the pupil looks out of the great circle alternately in one direction and in the other.

Plate 14 - Rhythm

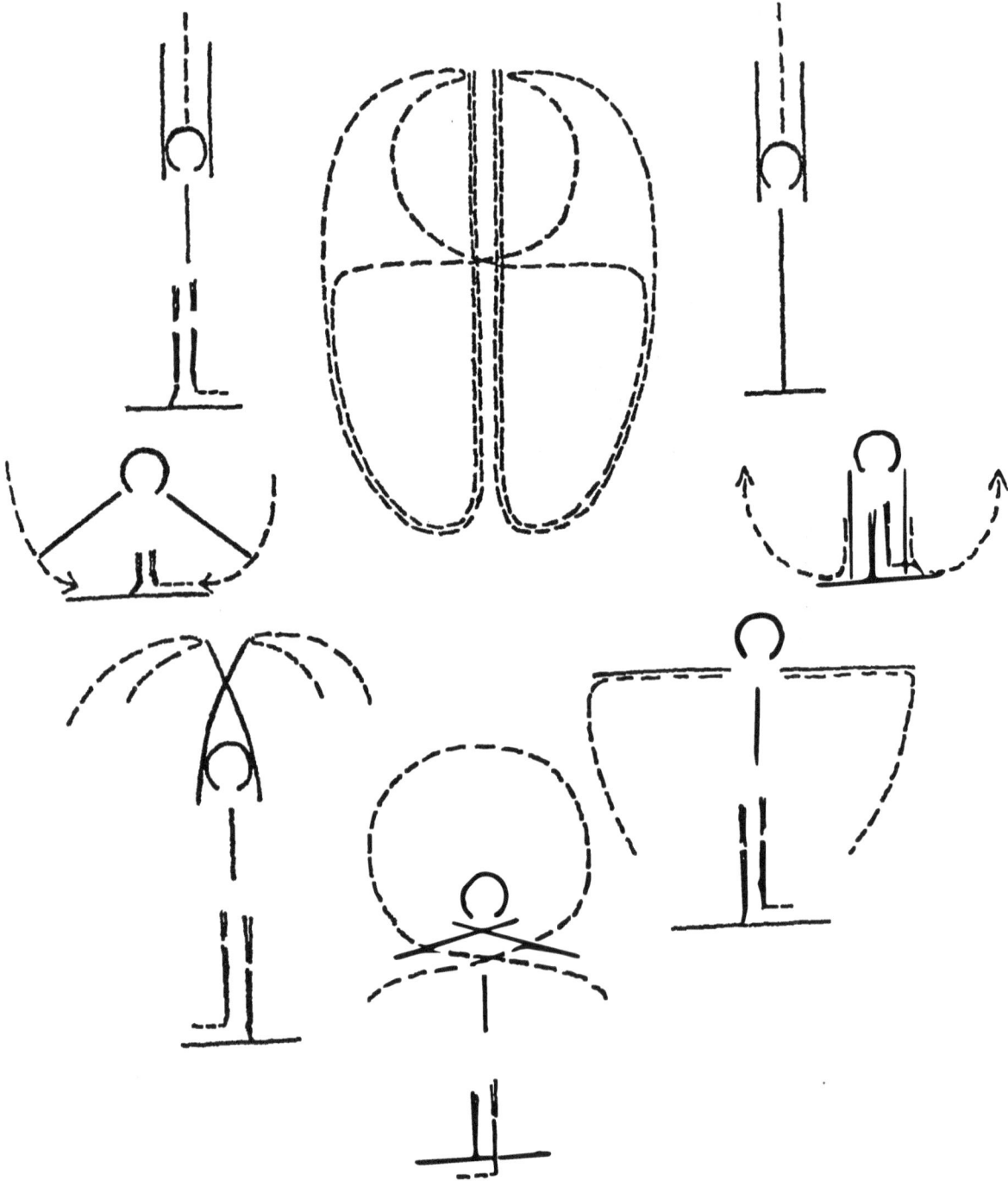

46

Rhythm streams freely through this whole exercise in great sweeping curves; a rhythm which carries pulse beat and breathing with it. Only in the moment of crossing is the rhythm slightly held; and here the pupil for an instant feels the resistance of the ground with his heels, as though, in this and in the crossing, to find strength for the following swing into the encircling sphere.

To set the feet one a little in front of the other, especially in the swing downward from height to depth, will give all the greater freedom of movement and also accords with the rather more three-dimensional character which this exercise has in comparison with the last.

A suitable name for this service would be "The Rhythm", for it is an archetypal picture of the very essence of rhythm. It is gymnastically of great value, and may be practiced with arms alone, singly or together, and at varying speeds; this may even be done in miniature with hands or fingers.

"The Jump into the Center of the Circle" demonstrates the powerful element of the will. This exercise reveals the fiery forces which rise up from the metabolic system.

"The Rhythm" is an expression of the forces which stream in from the periphery to the center and out again.

"The Triangle" is a picture of the formative forces proceeding from the head, - from the apex. This triad of exercises relates to thinking, feeling and willing in man, picturing his threefold organism, - head, chest and limb systems, (nerve-sense, rhythmic and metabolic systems). The three systems merge into one another, just as thinking, feeling and willing are interrelated, though each has its own center and derives its name therefrom. Similarly, we speak of the upper, middle and lower man.

The development of these three does not run parallel throughout childhood and youth.

During his first seven years, it is predominantly the forces radiating from the head which work formatively throughout the whole organism of the child.

In the second seven years, the forces which stream in and out between periphery and center, in the breathing and blood circulation, play an especially harmonious role, their rhythms bringing vitality, balance and therefore healing.

The third seven years is the time when the limb system is powerfully activated by the forces received through the metabolism. These forces may greatly strengthen the physical organism, but they may also overwhelm man.

Every gymnastic exercise contains within it, though in varying degrees, these three aspects, each of which may constitute an exercise complete in itself, although the three are really inseparable. It is only this threefold principle - a trinity - which can speak to the whole being of the child, so that consciously or unconsciously, through his thinking, feeling and willing, he feels himself addressed. In form and rhythm and in the measure of bodily force it calls for, each exercise, both as a whole and in its parts, must be true to the ideal picture of man which every healthy, uncorrupted human being bears within him. This was revealed in the exercises so far described and will be also in the ones to follow. (Note: Indications concerning tha nature of the human being are base on Rudolf Steiner's investigations published in his books and lectures.)

The Age of Puberty

The Fall into Space

After the spring into the center of the circle, which received into itself the forces of the heights, the pupil stands like a five-pointed star; the center his breast and the upward pointing ray his head. The power of the heights should here be felt with a spiraling quality. A pendulum swing leads breadth back to the vertical position, to height.

The force engendered by this swing to height is accumulated and dammed up in tension when the pupil clenches his fists above his head. Using the force thus pent up in his body, he overstretches upward, away from the form ground beneath his feet, and in overstretching, loses his balanced poise between heights and depths. Top-heavy, he falls forward.

The fall as such would quickly render man insensible and put an end to all movement, as with a tree that has been felled. This fall, an outcome of exaggerated height, is now caught up by a long step forward. The uplifted arms which, using the force that was dammed up in the clenched fists, have stretched the body to the utmost, now let go of the heights. They release themselves and the whole body from tension and, crossing and uncrossing as they go*, fall through the depths and spread out into width.** They carry the body through the depths and, after the forward step, bring it up into an inclined plane, endowing it once more with a state of balance in this plane. At the same time they re-enliven the body with rhythmic power.

Having been bound to one dimension by the constricted movement to height, the pupil, in falling, has attained three-dimensional space, and in doing so has placed himself under the severe restraint of gravity. With his arms after the fall he seeks the widths, and with his look forward goal, in order once more to gain a hold and orientate himself anew in space. Thanks to the free, swinging power of the arms, he is able to regain the heights, the vertical dimension.

If it were simply a matter of standing up again from the fallen position, nothing of significance would have happened gymnastically; it would be like standing a fallen tree up on its end again. It is however a question of endeavoring to find a new, changed relationship between the forces of the upward-striving human being and those of the earth which draw him down.

Just as in the fall he reached the third dimension at the cost of the first, height, which he divided into two as he let go of it; so now he must try, in attaining the heights once more, to re-establish three-dimensional space as a unity. Now he must achieve his standing position in such a way that it is woven through and filled with the living forces of space. Only then will the fall have been overcome gymnastically.

---

* Crossing with open hands in front of the chest during the fall; uncrossing again below in the transition from fall to rise.
** Palms face downward

48

Plate 15 The Fall into Space

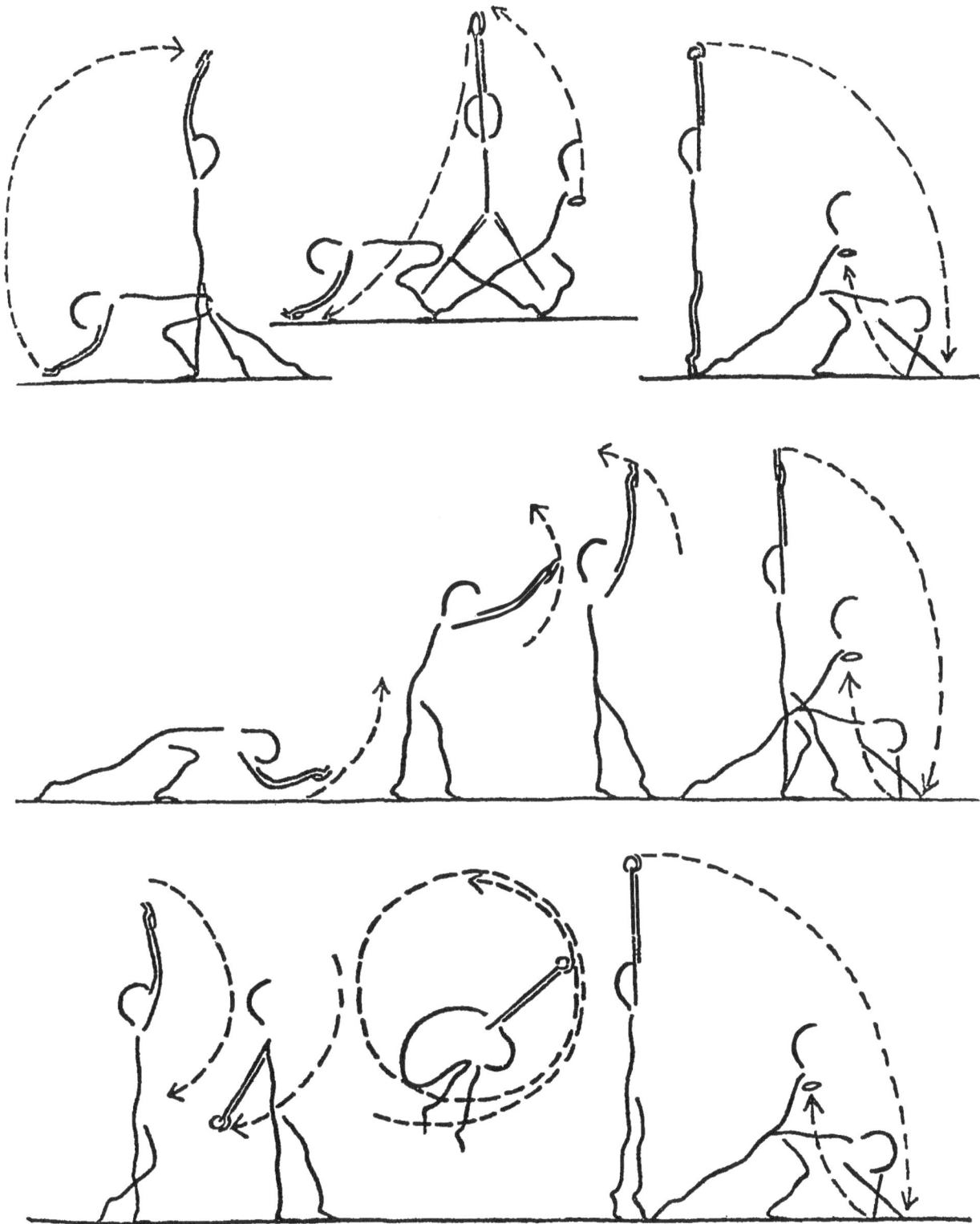

Using the force in his freely poised arms, the pupil swings himself up from the inclined plane, on the basis of the long step forward.* High above this base, as though in a pivotal point, he makes a quick turn through 180 degrees, dissolving the wide span of his arms, passing through the whole of the encircling sphere, through width and depth into the forward dimension, catching his body up again and raising it to height.** What was the rear leg during the fall forward is now the one supporting the body's weight, while the other is free to move. The freedom of balance which is thus achieved is no longer simply given by the dimensions of space as such, but is determined by the human form itself.

"I stand upright, firmly on the ground, one foot ready for a forward step."

The best position from which to begin the exercise as here described is with feet apart and arms outspread sideways. The teacher may accompany the exercise by saying the following:**

"Stand wide, with outspread arms.	Stretch up to...
Swing	Fall;
To height	And
Stem,	Turn
	To height."

---

* The upward swing of the arms on the basis of the long step results in the feet leaving the floor; that is to say, the upward rise of the arms draws the body upward in a spring. Thus the quick turn takes place as though in the air. This is made clear in the description of the leap on page 27 which corresponds to it.

** Here the palms of the hands are turned upward; the movement catches up the fall after the turn. The arms, in rising, draw the whole form into the upright position again. The quiet standing position is then reached with slightly best arms and hands, palms facing backward, while simultaneously - for the first time in the sequence of exercises - one foot is free to take a step.

** The exercise on page 16 now appears again as an introduction. There, it was "grow out over height into width", here "height" is exaggerated and the outcome is a fall. Bothmer often did the exercise without fists, but simply over-reaching upward. The spoken accompaniment might then be:

Jump into breadth	To height	Fall	Jump into Height	Rise	
Swing	Over-reach to	Rise in the Depth	Turn - Fall	Rise	To height

50

The pivoting turn divides the whole, stage by stage, into contrasting movement pictures which are of considerable significance.

On the one side there is great physical tension, answered by the fall where the release is almost tantamount to a condition of swooning. In this movement, yielding to gravity, the closed unity of height is divided into the duality of right and left; from this arises width.

On the other side there is a smooth rhythm, with no contrasting tensions and relaxations. There is conscious control of the space-forming aspect of the movement, in accordance with the true measure of man, whereby, instead of stretching up physically, man rises to his full human stature. And there is a drawing together of the parts to create a whole once more. On one side power is lost, to be received again on the other.

First Continuation through Swing

(Plate 15)

The first, elementary form of the fall through over-reaching to height, and its recovery, is capable of being developed further, leading to new and interesting variations of the same movement.

One leg bears the weight of the body and maintains a power of resistance to gravity; the other is free to take a step, forward or backward. Repetition of the whole movement follows as the free leg comes up from behind in the rise from the fall. the new movement links on with this, uniting with the forward and upward movement of the arms.

If the pupil follows the power of the movement in which the arms lead forward and upward, he may simply be carried on, or he may transform the fall into a light and widely swinging rhythm. The interplay between human force of gravity is then led over each time at the pivoting turn into an even movement going forwards and backwards of a pendulum and with a rhythm akin to that of the breathing.

Coming up out of the fall, the pupil takes a light resilient step forward and setting the other foot forward as though to take a second*, he swings it far back behind him**. At the same time, the arms, crossing and then spreading out to width, swing the body - as with the fall - forward into the inclined plane. Height is then regained as before, through the pivoting turn. The sequence of movements may be continued indefinitely.

The swinging movement of the outspread arms which always follows the fall, giving the upward impulse which lifts the movement into the pivoting turn, may be enhanced and repeated before the actual turn is made. The arms may then swing so high that the backs of the hands meet and touch and also so low that the fingers touch the ground.*

"	High, low
Stretch up to	And
Fall -	Turn
High, low,	to height."

---

* During this step and a half, the palms of the hands are turned forward. As the toe is set forward, arms, hands and fingertips reach height.
** The supporting foot accompanies this with a light resilient jump.
* Here the upward swing is to be identified entirely with an upward jump. As the arms swing low, the rear foot slips far back.

Second Continuation through Jump

(Plate 15)

Instead of following the pull of the movement forward and upward after the pivoting turn and thus remaining freely poised amid the place of forces, the movement may become congested and harden again in height. This tendency to harden upward in resistance, can be developed gymnastically, leading to an exercise opposite in character to the one just described.

To stress the moment of resistance at the end of the rising movement, the free foot treads firmly backward while the arms are thrust forward and downward and back. The fists are clenched, to enhance the tension which now grips the whole body. The movement is liberated again by a high leap forward,** accompanied and activated by a strong circling movement of the arms. But this leap brings freedom only for a moment, ending in the position of tension upward to height which brought about the fall in the first place. The outcome, therefore, is the fall again, which can again be caught up in the inclined plane. The solution to this is the pivoting turn, with the subsequent rise upward to the vertical. The whole sequence of movements may be repeated indefinitely.

Throughout these transformations, the basic exercise retains its character, always resulting in the experience of widening out into space, and laying emphasis all the while on polar opposite qualities in movement. The contrasting pictures of the fall and the recovery from it are divided by the pivoting turn; there is separation on one side and fusion on the other; the picture of gravity, on the one, and of its opposing force on the other; the way in which the will be can be caught and held in the limb-system, while a balancing, healing force works in the rhythmic system. But not only this. The polarities are united in the fulcrum, the space-forming consciousness of man, through which in the final outcome, the overcoming of the fall, the new "I stand" is achieved every time.

The two polarities, the will, sometimes rampages, and the rhythm with its calming action, are both given due and worthy expression in these two variations of the exercise, and they reveal the contrast of man and woman. In spite of their contrasts in dynamic force, they have the same rhythmic beat, so that they can be practiced together. To do this, very much enriches the gymnastic work, especially in mixed classes.

The rhythm common to these two variations of the fall is as follows:

First variation:

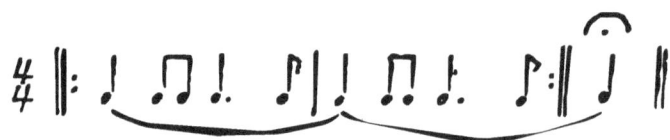

Second variation:

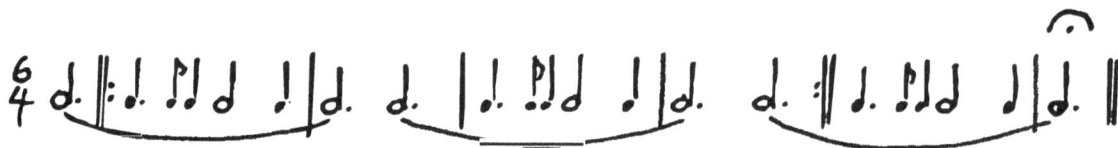

** This leap is described on page 85. It is a double leap and the arms almost describe two circles. The rising movement of the arms, repeated twice, enhances the upward lift of the spring. Fists are opened again in the outspread movement of the arms which follows.

If both variations are to be performed at the same time, their rhythms may be brought together in two ways:

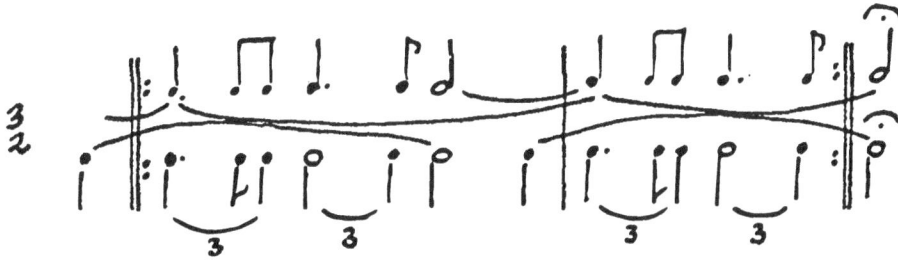

If the two variations are practiced together, it is good to unite them at the end and close with the form and rhythm of the first variation, letting the movement come to an end in the slower rhythm. The transition can equally well be made from the second variation.* This exercise, together with what has gone before, belongs to the time of puberty. Throughout the rest of the upper school the classes will however continue to work at it and bring it to perfection.

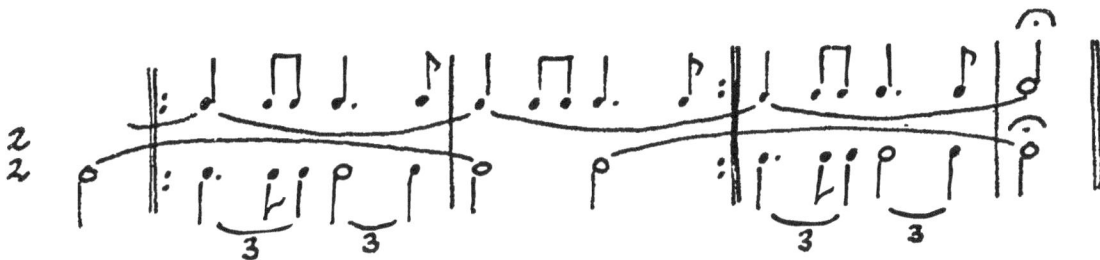

---

* The difference in the two rhythms is also revealed spatially. Just as in time, the first variation takes place twice while the second one happens once, so the second variation takes up more space. The double step (spring-plus-fall) of the second variation contrasts with the small backward and forward steps of the first.

After the Age of Puberty

The Fall into the Point

The "Fall into the inclined plane and the recovery", including as it does the decisive step across the threshold of the third dimension - the fall into space, - is the natural culmination of the gymnastic training in the lower school.

The "Vertical Fall", in common with this earlier exercise, takes its start from the heights. It may be regarded as the fall into a point, coming about through relinquishing height as a result of the one-sided influence of sheer weight and gravity. It involves the most extreme degree of bodily surrender and collapse.

As an example of what happens in the vertical fall, I hold my arm straight up and then suddenly withdraw all the strength from it. It falls directly. If I were to do the same with the force which keeps my body upright, all my joints would give way, allowing the body to collapse in a heap on the ground.

This vertical fall, left to itself, is final; but it can be caught up in movement. One foot is brought forward, to save the body from being jolted and from actually crashing to the ground, and the arms are saved by bending them. This movement of foot and arm implies the use of the last remaining ounce of force left to counteract the impotence of the fall. The fall from exaggerated height ended with the body spread out in a wide cross in the inclined plane, whereas after the vertical fall the limbs are bent double and the body rounded to a small sphere, to a point. Space is lost.

From this dead point, the body, without strength or breath, will not so easily rise up again. In order to regain space and rhythm, the pupil reaches into space with his arms, taking at the same time a tentative step forward. The arms, reaching for space, move in a circle,* at first almost to the ground and then forward and upward, closing the circle just in front of the shoulders. This movement in pure rhythm, - the spatial picture of drawing a deep breath.

The expanding of the sphere, drawing together at the close, gives the power which brings the body up; it rises out of the center** with yet another step forward. The arms accompany this steep rise to the heights.

With this, however, neither space nor a new state of balance is achieved. The exaggerated and overstressed movement to height lacks a stable footing. This footing is found when the weight of the body is brought down resolutely on the backward foot, with a firm tread, which withstands the pressure, while simultaneously the arms are pressed down from above, forward into the horizontal. The wrists bend, so that the palms face forward. The wrists bend, so that the palms face forward. The hands still point to height, and the arms, stretched and taut, reveal the strong force of resistance.

The tension which thus comes about between forward and backward is resolved in a forward step; this parts the resistance and opens out the way forward. Then follows the release of the arms out of the horizontal balance to the resting position.

---

* Hands move parallel to one another.
** With a powerful spring, which is so steep that the accompanying step amounts really only to a change of feet.

54

Plate 16 – The Fall into the point

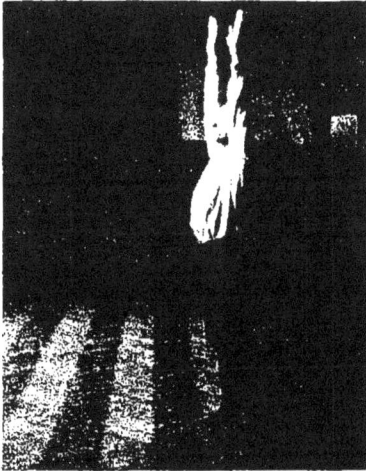

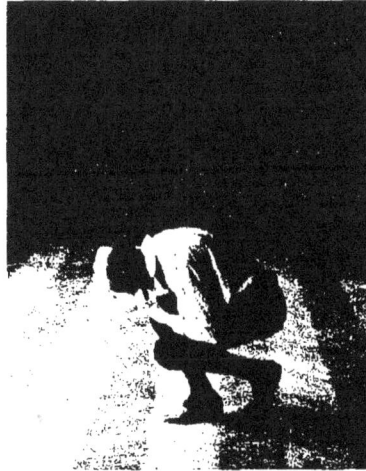

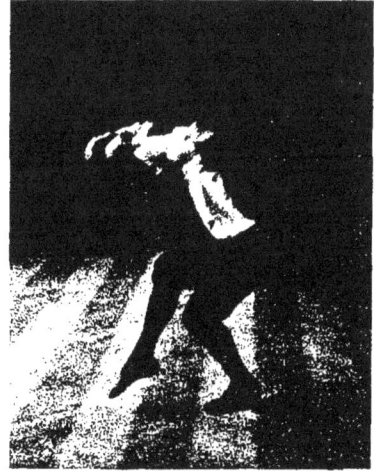

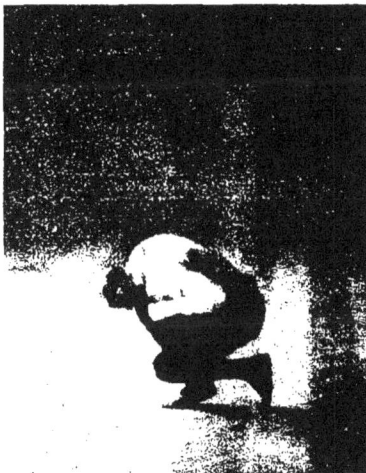

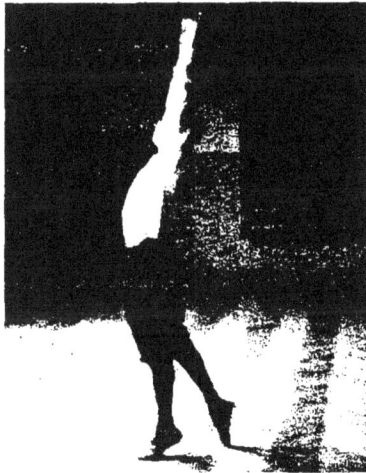

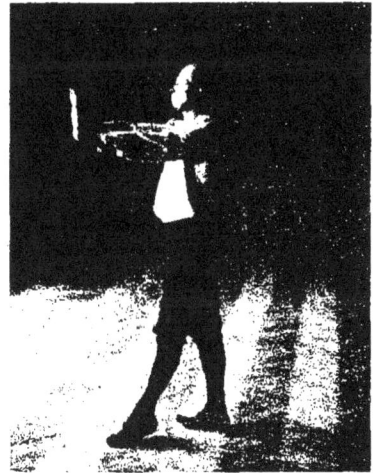

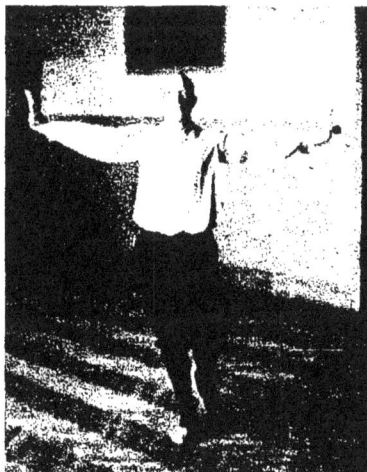

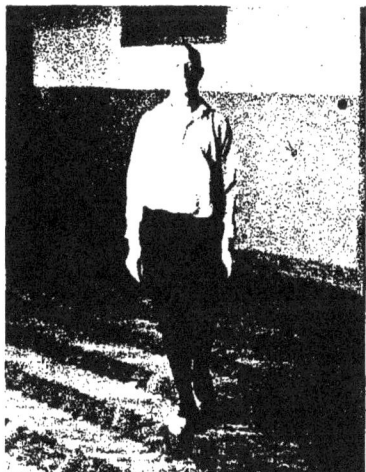

Now at last the new condition of equilibrium is achieved. This state of balance is no longer subject to the fall and freedom to step forward and backward is inherent in it.

Thus is the seal of three-dimensionality imprinted upon space by the strength and stature of man; the vertical has been regained in rising upright; the breadth in parting the resistance; the forward vision and movement towards a goal have been made free.

"I stand, upright in the three dimensions, free to take a step towards my goal."

The fall is overcome.

Continuation

This readiness to take a step makes possible a new contraction, - not downward, as before in the collapse from height, but towards the middle region, supported by the leg which is standing on the ground. The head and the free leg come together from above and below, while the arms and hands, first reaching out - as they did after the fall - with a rounded movement forward into space, are then brought close together in front of the chest. Even the supporting leg plays its part in this movement towards the middle, for it is acting as a strut, holding the body upward. Then, pushing energetically from the ground with the free leg and thus taking another step forward, the pupil springs out of the contracted position upward again to height.

This time height, springing as it has done from the middle region, does not need to become consolidated by meeting with resistance and in a backward tread, as was the case after the fall. Rather does it seek to be freely sustained by kindred forces in the wide expanse. It swings from its highest point, carried by the supporting foot, into a cross in the horizontal plane; the eyes look forward, arms cross over and then spread out; the other leg is freely poised behind. This is a real test of balance. It comes temporarily to rest simply by standing erect on the supporting leg. But only through a renewed drawing inward of the arms, which are then thrust forward, while the free foot receives the weight of the body firmly backward, is the movement consolidated in meeting with resistance. Then, with a forward step, resistance is parted in the balance to the horizontal and resolved.

Out of the original threefold movement of "spring, tread and step" (height, backward and forward), there has now arisen the fourfold movement, spring, swing, tread and step (height, width, backward, forward).

The quaternary also establishes the relation to the dynamics of the four elements, that are at work in the human body:

> Fire, which flames to the heights,
> Air, which flows to and from the widths,
> Earth, which is firmly resistant,
> Water, which glides and spreads out.

Plate 17- The fall into the point - Continuation

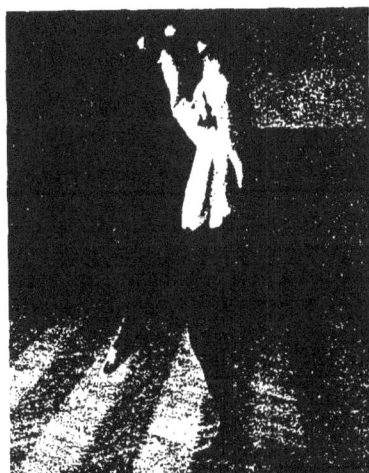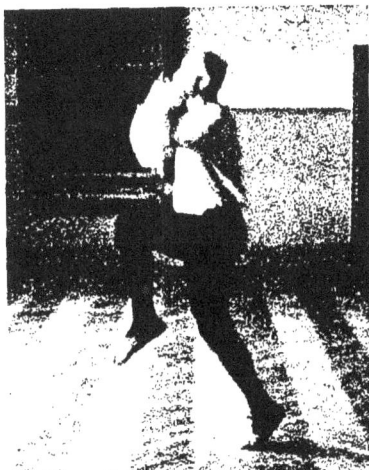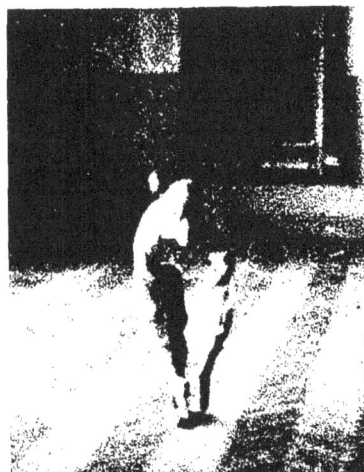

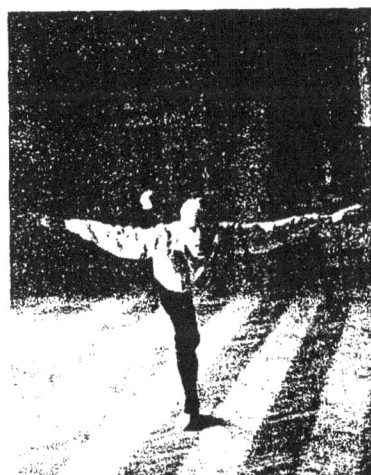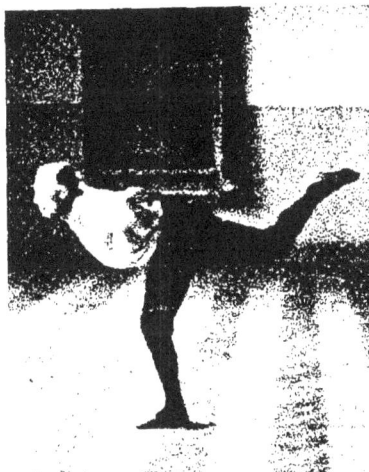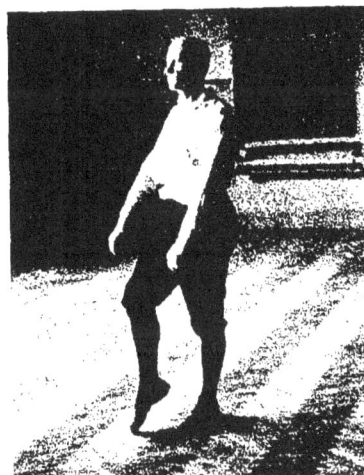

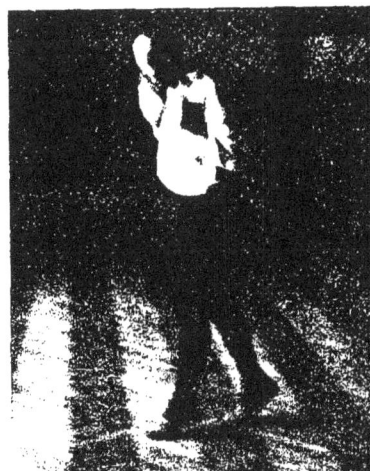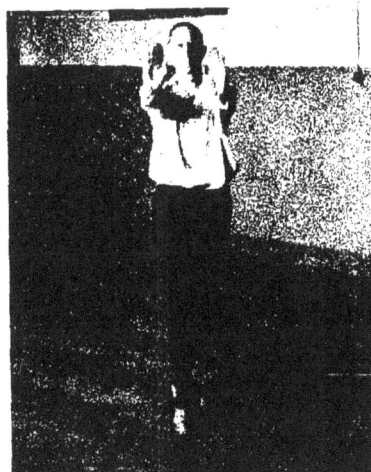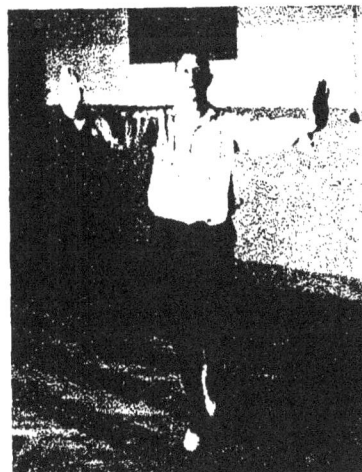

Walking or Stepping

Walking, or stepping, is gymnastically the synthesis of these four elements of movement; it united them all. The dramatic development of the vertical fall flows over at last into a forward stepping movement; the arms are again raised from the resting position to make the wide forward-reaching circling movement towards the center, then, drawing together, they are thrust out sideways in the horizontal, while the free foot either comes forward for a step or treads firmly to the ground behind, thus releasing the other foot.

Plate 18

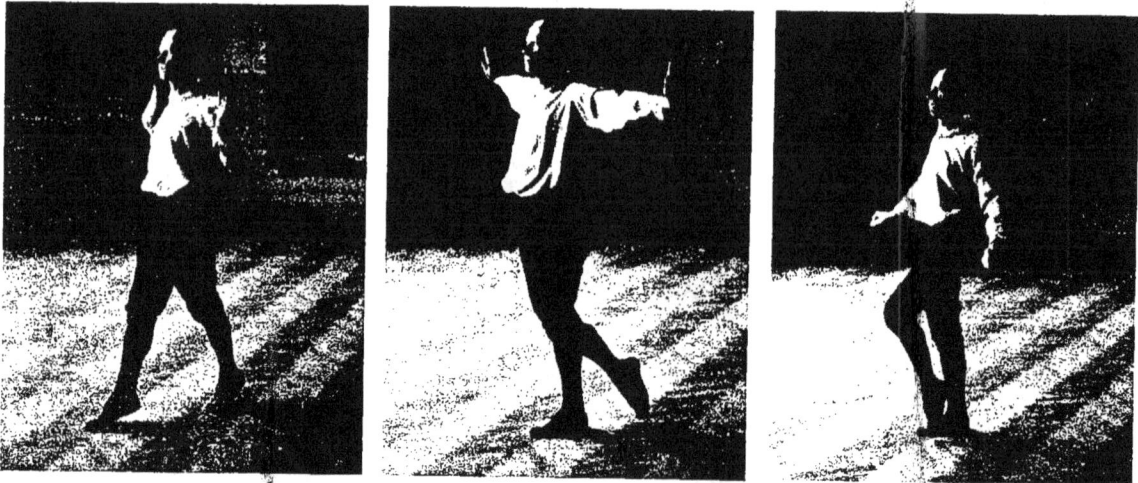

The pupil continues to walk, forward or backward, moving through the resistance as through an alley, the walls of which are built up on either side by the upturned palms of the hands, as the arms are pushed out sideways in the horizontal. He walks along with smooth flowing step, the rhythm of which is given by the arms in drawing together, pushing, pressing sideways and releasing

The eyes are directed immutably forward to the aim or goal.

In the fall from exaggerated height into the inclined plane, the recovery, after the turn, was made up by an upward movement filled with the active forces of the wide expanse. Here, there were richer possibilities of movement, even in the fall itself with its variations.

The vertical fall into the point is uniform. All the more manifold and rich is the play of forces in the recovery. This exercise lays more emphasis on the experience of bodily strength. Rhythm is at first less in evidence; the actual dimension-forming forces of space are predominant. But the aim of the whole - an aim worth striving for - is to imbue these space-forming forces with rhythm; more and more to develop the dynamic forces inherent in the sudden jump, the upward rise, the thrust, the gliding movement, in spring, swing, tread and step, in drawing together and releasing. All are included in a unified, continuous movement, and never for a moment must the thread of continuity be lost or broken.

It would be quite wrong simply to ascribe movements or sheer bodily strength to the man and rhythmical movements to the woman. Rhythm is no less important for the man, protecting him from

58

becoming hardened and mechanical, than is the exercising of bodily power for the woman. In some exercises, however, the man especially will feel his bodily powers called forth, others will appeal to the woman's more rhythmical nature. Every exercise is fully suited to both sexes and necessary for their right development.

Between the two "Falls" lies the actual threshold of puberty; it is, both gymnastically and in childhood development, the most incisive moment, marking the end of an educational period and the beginning of a time of manifold growth and realization in the field of gymnastics.

Rhythm of two interlacing Circles - Frontal Plane

The walking exercise which was born out of the vertical fall and its recovery, laid emphasis on bodily strength through the sideways movement of the arms.

A walking exercise, in which harmoniously synchronized movement of the upper and lower parts of the body are enhanced and developed into a widely swinging rhythm, is derived from the interplay of two circles. It may begin either simply by crossing the arms behind the back, or it may be led out of the crossing which occurs in the "Re-entrant Triangle".*

In that exercise the arms, crossed at the nape of the neck in the last position of resistance, were opened up in the beginning of a circular movement. Now the arms continue on down in this circle until they are crossed once more; this time the backs of the flat hands touch the middle of the back. At the same time, one foot is released from the ground and brought forward in readiness for a step.

The arms then uncross downward, moving in a widely spanned circle; this movement takes place with a deep bend of the knees, so that the lowest point of the circle reaches to the heel of the supporting foot, after which the arms, continuing to rise in the circle, bear the body up until they cross and close the circle again between the shoulder-blades. While this is happening, the step is continued smoothly, until the weight of the body has been transferred to the other foot.

Then, while the arms uncross again above and return in a smaller circle to the lower crossing point, the free foot comes forward, ready for another step.* (26)

A simple, quiet rhythm is thus developed between the two circles, a large circle created from below upward and a smaller one from above downward. This interplay is carried forward by the smooth stepping movement until the rhythm is brought to rest in the upright standing position. Following the strong, energetic re-entrant triangle exercise, this quiet circling rhythm has a harmonious influence.

---

* From the standing position the exercise is begun by lifting the arms sideways and up to cross at the nape of the neck.
* It would also be possible to make the steps so that the free foot is set forward as the arms come to the crossing, while the weight comes forward on this foot as the arms uncross again. Compare with this the "Twofold eight" in its simplified form (page 62) and the "Walking with circling arms" (page 66)

Plate 19

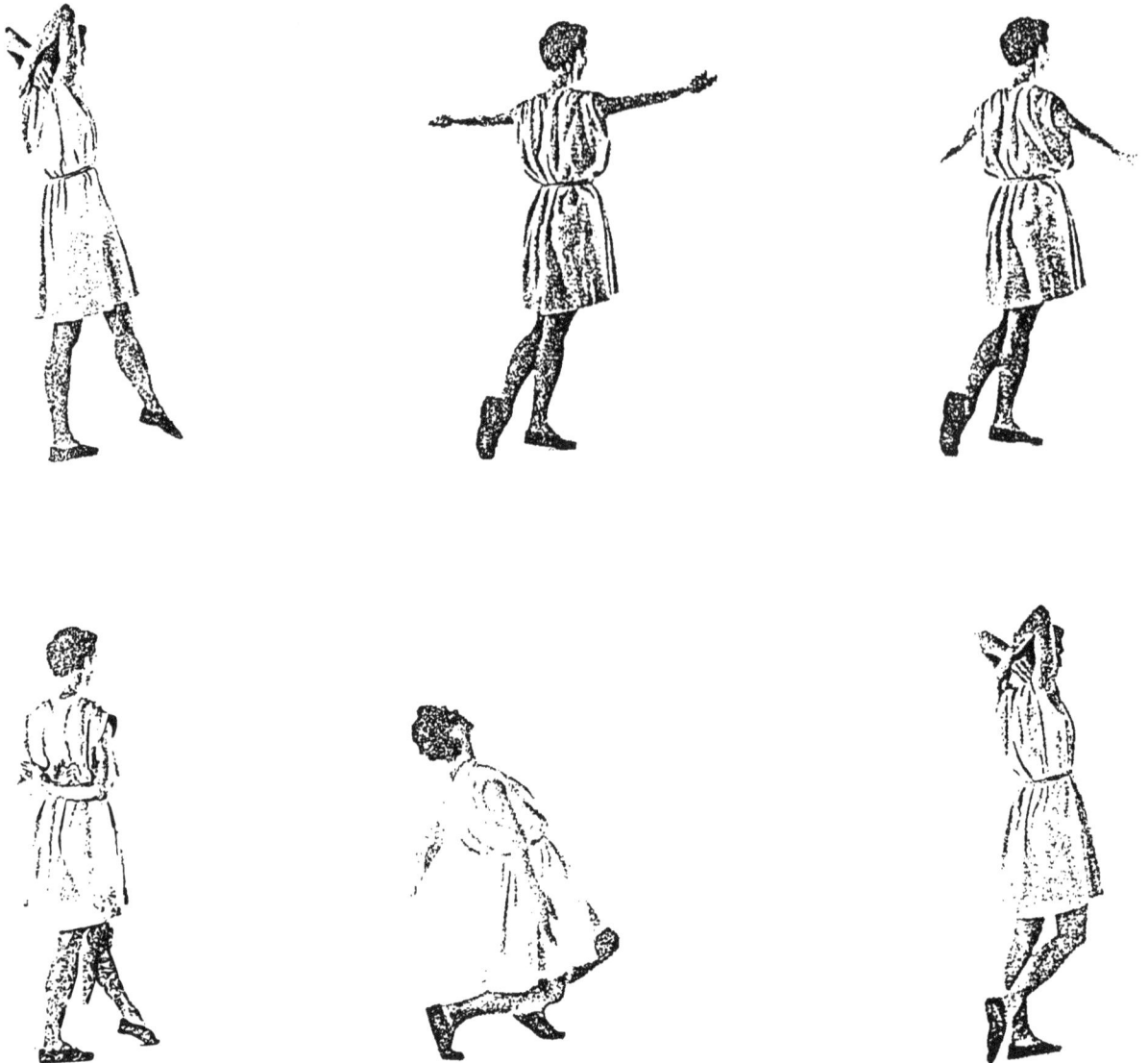

The activated Fall

(See Plate 20)

The activated fall, or lunge, in contrast to the mere fall, is a deliberate movement in which the fall is accelerated by the individual's own power . It is developed out of the movement which exaggerates height; one foot is set to take a step and the clenched fists congest the movement and over-reach to the utmost in height. Upheld by the supporting leg, height is then plunged in a steep forward and downward swing, until the head is below and the fists above again. The free leg is lifted from in front and set far back, giving free play to the movement and sustaining it like a buttress from behind.

The fists have moved in a spiral which includes the head and trunk, thus giving rise to a tremendous congestion of forces. Release follows in a forceful upward movement back to height, which is introduced by a quiet drawing together movement, upward towards the middle. With a strong downward tread of the free leg, the spiral unwinds again swiftly, releasing the clenched hands and ending in a circling movement of the arms. With this movement the step, which was begun in the deliberate fall, is completed.

The movement resolving the activated fall may go over once more into the congested exaggeration of height, to be followed again by the fall and the ascent as before.

From the vertical fall onward, every exercise is really a dramatically graduated step - a kind of walking movement; through the repetition, a certain distance is covered rhythmically, as is the case in walking. This expresses the attainment of conscious control over the very essence of the third dimension.

Plate 20 – The activated fall

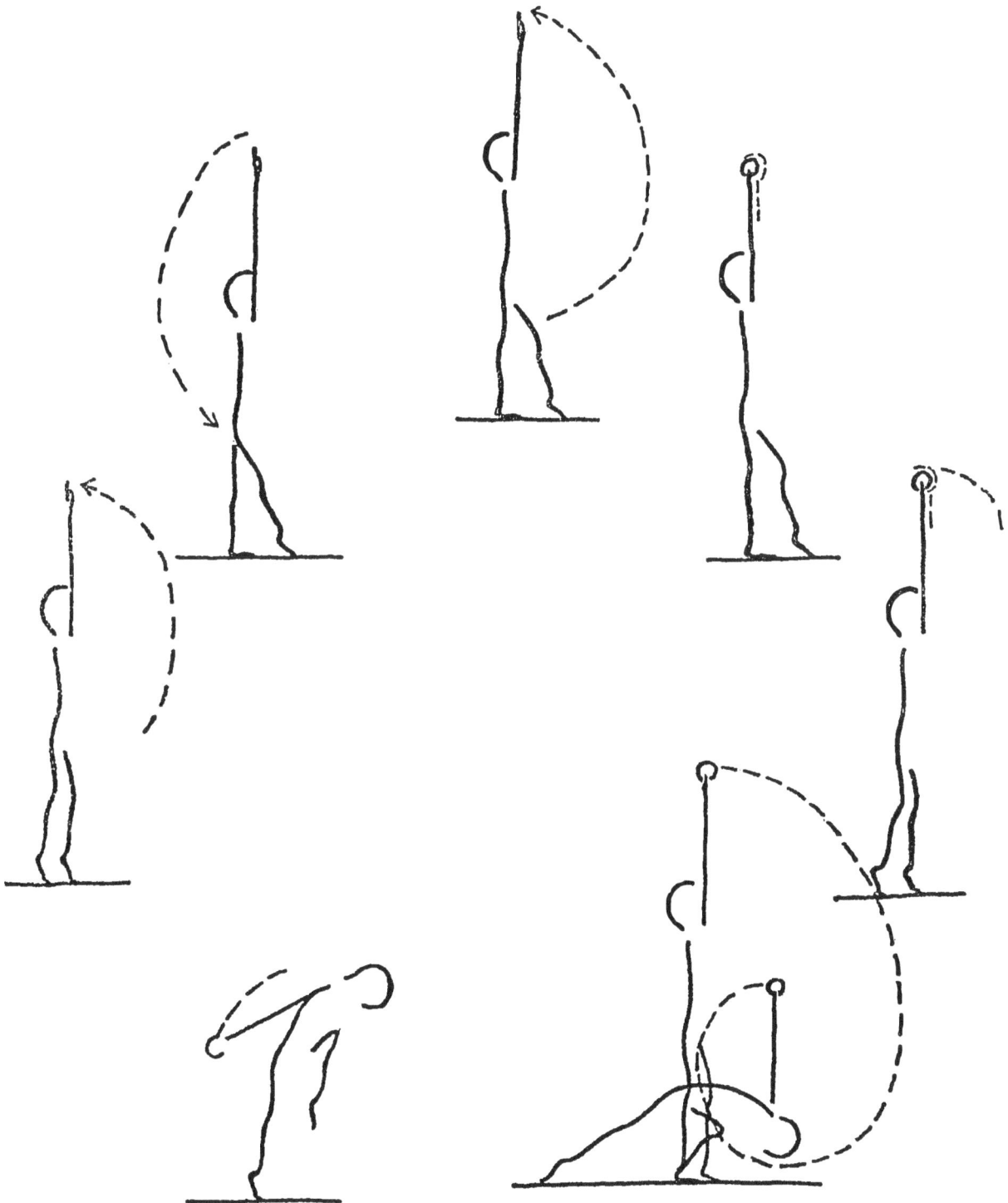

The Whirl or Vortex

(See Plate 21)

Quite another kind of tension comes about when height is congested downward. The supporting leg bends under the pressure from above; the free foot, which has been set ready for a step, makes room by sliding forward. When the pressure becomes so strong that balance is endangered, it will be released by a strong sweep of the arms from heights down through depths, whereby, between the pressure from above and the congestion from below, they are set moving in a whirl or vortex, spiraling around the horizontal. The movement restores the balance of the body by raising it to the vertical and then comes to rest in the horizontal. Not until the arms are led over from width to height in the final movement to the vertical, is the step, which was prepared at the beginning, completed. Then a new step is prepared.

Plate 21

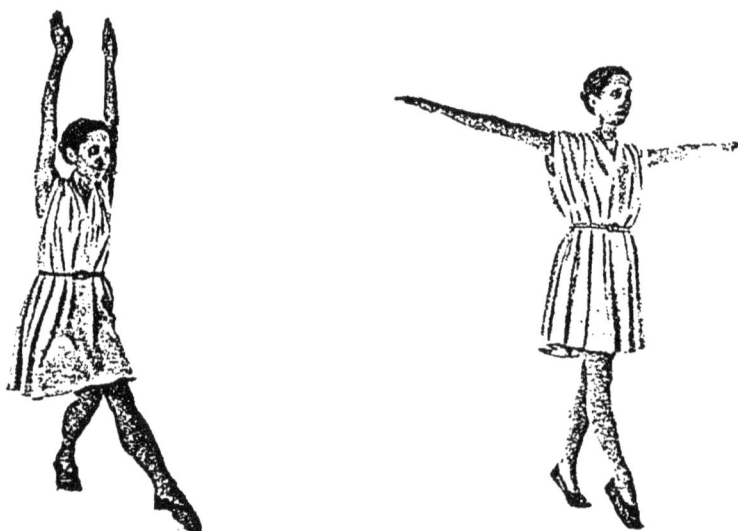

Twofold Eight

If the arms reaching to height, instead of being together, are one behind the other, palms facing, but in a plane, and if this height id then pressed down towards depth, balance will not be restored by a sideways spiraling movement of the arms around the horizontal axis, but by a movement in which the arms follow one another in the plane of symmetry. As though on the cutting edge of a knife, the arms move down in this vertical plane, making their way forward and to the depths, and passing close by the body, both on the same side. As they move up behind, towards the horizontal, they slowly bring the body up. They then no longer remain in the same plane and are moving beside one another when they pass through the horizontal plane behind the body, making a strange play of lines and angles as they do so. Until now, one leg has carried all the weight. The free leg had at first given in to the downward pressure by sliding forward; now it comes back again as the movement lifts to the horizontal.

While the arms lead the movement on up to height, they move again into the same plane, one behind the other, and passing the uppermost point, they continue their way down on the other side of the body. With this, one hand takes over the lead from the other.

62

Each time the movement passes up through the horizontal behind the body, the weight goes over from one leg to the other. Eyes may either follow the movement of the arms and the play of the hands, or they may remain directed forward.

It is the rhythm of two interlacing figures-of-eight each with a smaller and a large loop inclining alternately on either side of the body from the apical point.

Plate 22

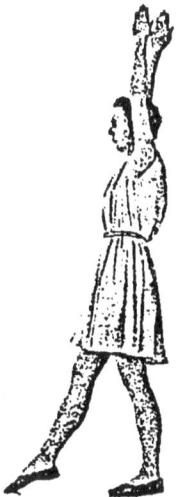

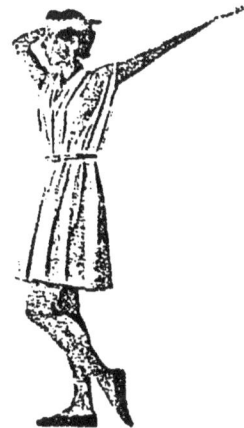

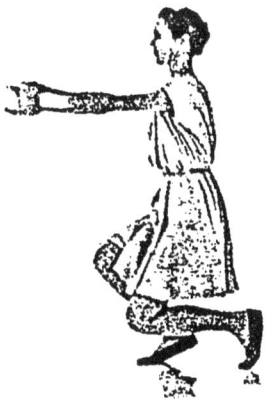

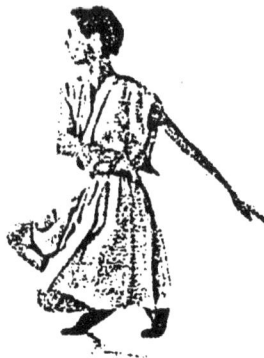

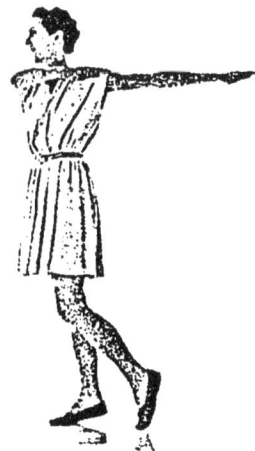

A simplification would be for the downward pressure to be sustained equally by both legs. Then the weight of the body will already pass over from one leg to the other during the left towards the horizontal. The free leg then follows. In this simpler form, the exercise may be done with many variations in the quality of dynamic force, from a quiet movement concentrating on the spatial form to a powerfully moving rhythm. This will start with a little jump and continue, remaining on the spot, feet alternating.

The character of the exercise, with its emphasis on the cutting movement in the plane of symmetry, remains unchanged.

The symmetry plane divides man, and through man space, into right and left; and it contains the aim or goal of forward movement. The symmetry plane gives the spatial direction of stepping and walking, of length, of the forward-backward dimension.

Most natural expression is given to the plane of symmetry in spear-throwing, in the shooting of the arrow from the bow, in the sword-stroke and the thrust of the lance; in all of these the dynamics of direction are at work. Spear-throwing is the most evident expression of the raying, radiating force, revealing the upright stature of man and belonging symbolically to him.

Bow and Arrow (See Plate 23)

Like an arrow from a bow, the spear shoots from the tension of the bowed body. This dynamic movement can be transformed into a gymnastic exercise closely resembling the throwing of a spear. In it the student is himself first bow and then arrow.

The archer stands in a quarter turn to the right; the right foot is set well back; the left shoulder, with outstretched arm and hand, and the eyes, are directed forward to the target. Then, as though putting an arrow to the bow, he puts the right hand to the left one. Allowing the outstretched, forward arm to act as resistance, he draws the right hand with clenched fist far back and downward behind him, bending his body to a spanned bow. Then, with a springing leap, the whole body follows this hand (opening) forward in the direction of the arrow, as though it were being shot from the bow. Thus, the archer is himself first bow, then arrow. After leaping forward, he seeks his balance again in the forward movement.

Plate 23

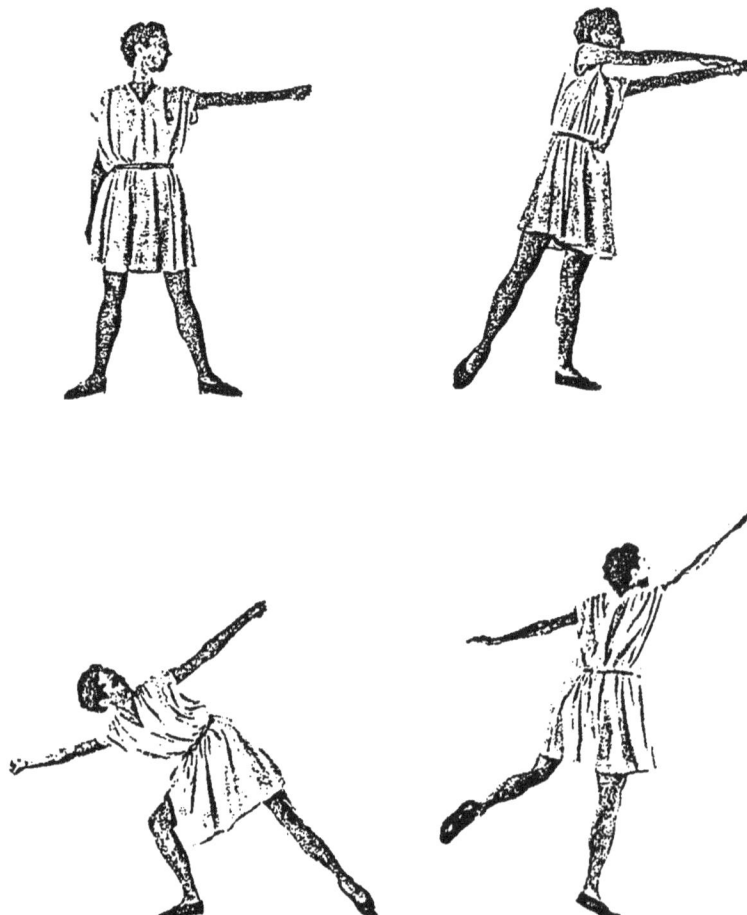

This exercise, which may be done alternately to right and left, is a picture of raying force. It appears again, transformed in a way which brings its nature clearly to manifestation, in the two exercises which may be called "the great horizontal" and "the great vertical".

Throwing the Discus

A rhythmical, circling force is involved in throwing the discus. The round disc is in direct contrast to the straight spear. The spear has a keen, sharp flight. The discus turns in flight, receiving its force from the wide swing, which is in effect a flat figure-of-eight spanned in a plane around the thrower and enhanced, in the turning step, to a circle. From this, the discus flies off tangentially, revolving round its own center.

The throw of the discus, (without the disc), may also be made into a gymnastic exercise. If a man stands upright, firmly on the ground, turning the body alternately to right and left and gradually accelerating the movement, his loosely swinging arms will begin to move in a sort of cone around him, which, as the arms are flung further and further out, widens and becomes a disc. The movement will be further enhanced if the student puts one foot forward and comes, through the continued circling movement, into a forward- and backward-swaying rhythm. Through the natural fall of the loosely hanging arms at the two points where the circles touch and change direction, the rhythmic movement assumes the form of a figure-of-eight. With a turning step, it can at the end be lead over to a spin, from which the throwing movement develops.

Plate 24

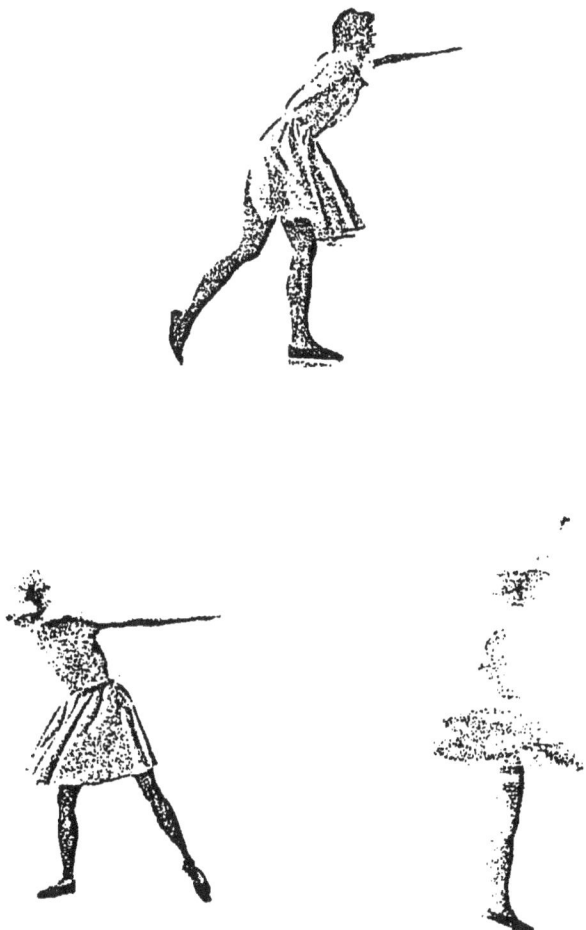

Walking with circling Arms

(See Table 25)

If in the gymnastic exercise the turning, flinging movement is slowed down to a quiet circling of the arms in the horizontal plane, a rhythm will arise which plays between expanding to the wide spaces and drawing together to the center; the movement is spanned out in a line to the greatest width and releasing from this, it spirals inward, drawing in towards the chest and behind the back.

This rhythm may be accompanied by walking with even, flowing steps. The great span into width gives the moment when the foot touches the ground, while during the inward and outward play of the spiral the free foot moves forward. This walking rhythm begins and ends in the widths.

It is clear that practiced purely as a gymnastic exercise, throwing the spear and throwing the discus have quite a different significance than if spear and discus are actually thrown. Without an object, the student experiences more consciously the realities underlying the movement, of the raying line in the spear-throw and the circling expansion into the wide spaces in the throw of the discus.

Movement directed to an Aim or Goal

(See Plate 26)

A gymnastic movement, which derives from the movement-motif of spear-throwing, brings the arms to the horizontal, emphasizing the direction of the goal in the forward-backward dimension, accompanied by a falling step or lunge, also in this dimension. This motif is capable of innumerable transformations before its possibilities for gymnastic movement are exhausted.

Consciously directing his will towards a goal, the student lunges, as though drawn forward by a magnet, catching himself up with arms extended horizontally, forward and backward. He would soon lose his balance and fall forward, if the force of direction alone were to continue to work. But at the moment of greatest tension, the forward movement has for an instant to pass through the vertical position. From there it is able to stream forward again with renewed force and with another falling step towards the goal. This intervention by the power of the vertical is necessary, because without it the forward movement, which only unites man and his aim in the sphere of instinct, would approach the bounds of what is permissible for man and would assume the characteristic quality of animal movement.

The vertical intervention may be enhanced to the extent of damming up the forward flow of movement, or it can be transformed and enriched through a temporary displacement of the goal itself.

Plate 25 – Walking with circling arms

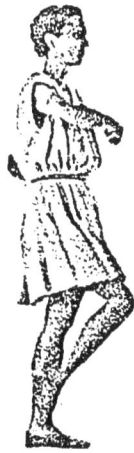

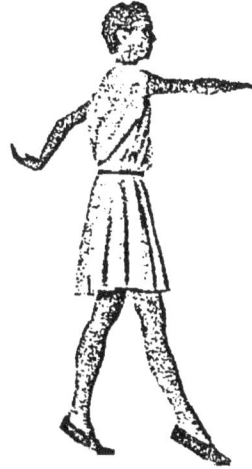

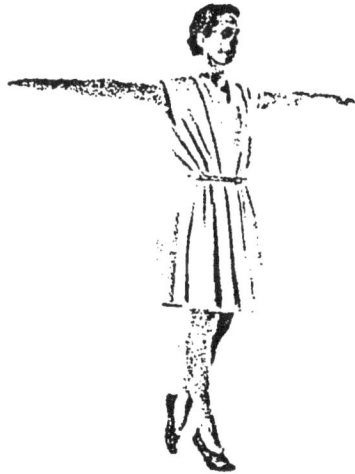

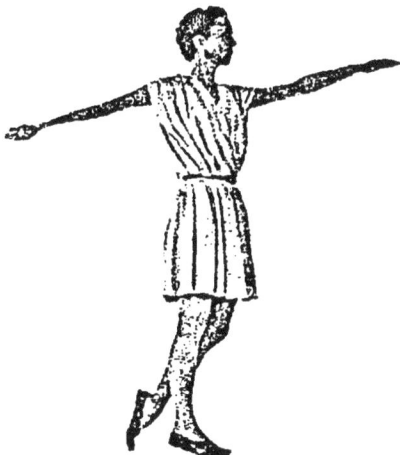

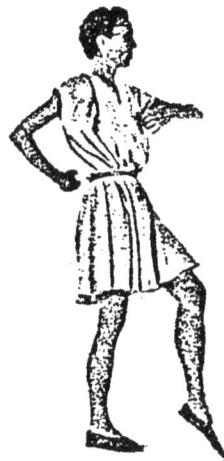

Plate 26 – Movement directed to a goal

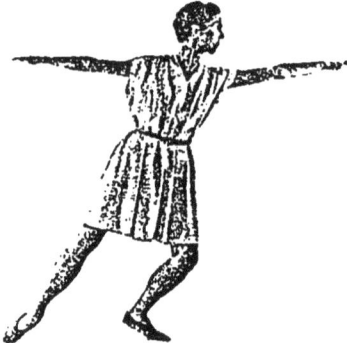

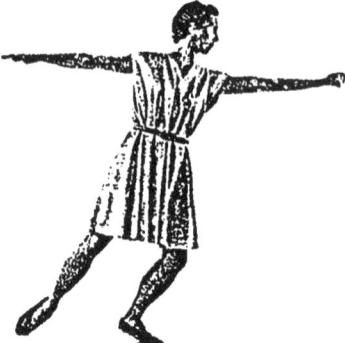

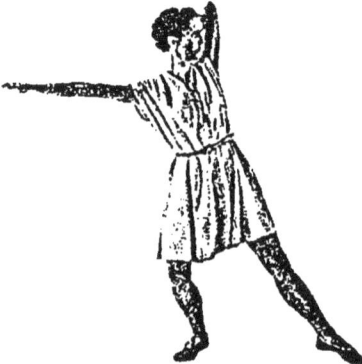

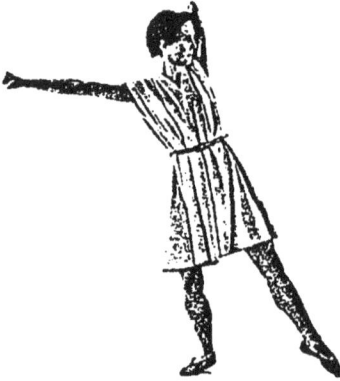

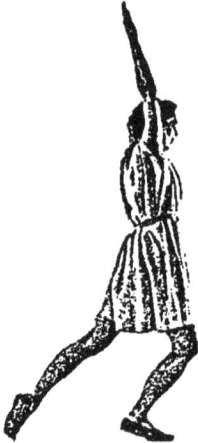

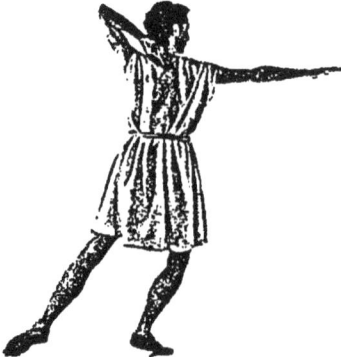

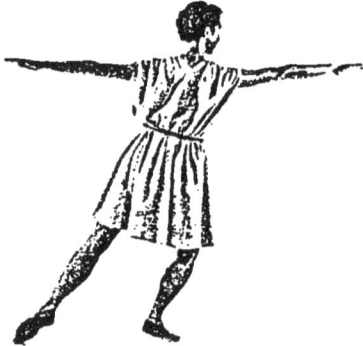

Just as the flow of water as it approaches a weir becomes congested and dammed up, then breaks, is thrown back, and then, uniting again with the onward-streaming force, throws itself against the obstacle, either to break through or overflow it; so now, gymnastically, the streaming will forces, flowing all one way in the direction of the goal, are dammed up precipitously. In the flow backward, they unite again with the stream coming from behind and, turning with another lunging movement towards the goal, they dive back into the forward-streaming flow of movement.

The force of the forward movement, reversed through the damming-up process, transfers the whole body backward,* and the arm which was pointing to the goal, seeking resistance, hits back into the nape of the neck. The free force of the backward-pointing arm then swings through depth to height, slinging the movement forward into another lunge. While this happens, the other hand remains at the nape of the neck, and the eyes look constantly forward.

Congestion of the movement may be effected either by clenching the fist of the forward hand, or by turning the flat palm upward, in which case, bending to make an effective hit backwards into the furrow between the shoulders, it then leads on to an open, throwing movement forward. After this forward slinging movement, both arms immerse themselves** in the horizontal once more and the play of forces begins anew.

Through this damming up process and its outcome, the student enhances the outer force of the forward movement, for in it the will is working predominantly in the physical forces of the body.

The movement may be enriched by further variations, in which the original goal and the direction towards or away from it is brought to consciousness still more strongly, while space is formed and imbued with living force:

The great Horizontal

(See Plate 27)

The goal moves its position, at first rising upward, and the student follows with his arms, which were outspread at first in the horizontal, forward-pointing direction. On the basis of the long step he took, he transfers his weight far back and down. Then the goal returns to the forward position and arms dip back again to the original direction, after which the student continues his way forward.

In this exercise, the whole body becomes like a balance with its swinging beam. It can either move up with the line of vision or it can swing against it; or it may do first one and then the other. It is like a deep breathing rhythm in space.

When the balance swings in the direction opposite to that taken by the line of vision, the weight of the body moves forward, the beam of the balance and the line of sight coming together in the zenith. Then the balance follows the line of sight onward through the whole sphere, until at last, turned backward, it finds the point on the horizon opposite to the one from which it started, having moved through a semicircle. Now the eyes are looking backward, while all the power of the body is striving forward. To continue forward from here, it is necessary as before, to pass for a moment through the vertical position in order to prepare for the new step; at the same time the eyes turn quickly in search of the original forward aim, and the rhythm can begin anew.

---

* The weight springs backward, from the forward foot to the backward one.
** One hand is opened again as it swings up, the other as it reaches to the horizontal backward; both reach the horizontal with palms upward.

Plate 27 – The great Horizontal

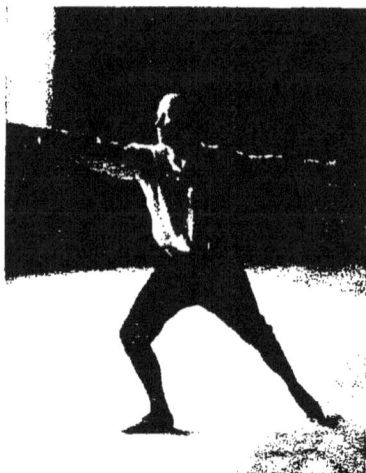

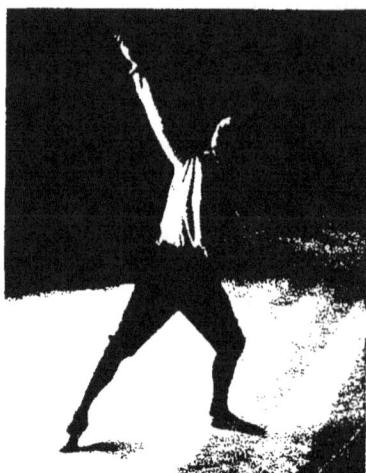

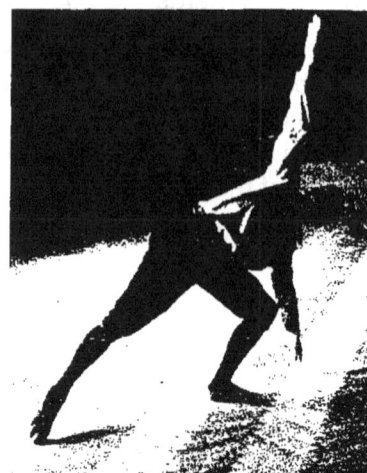

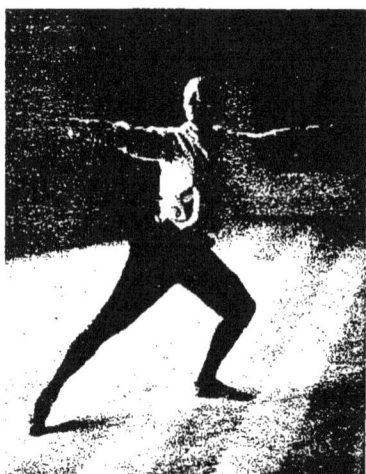

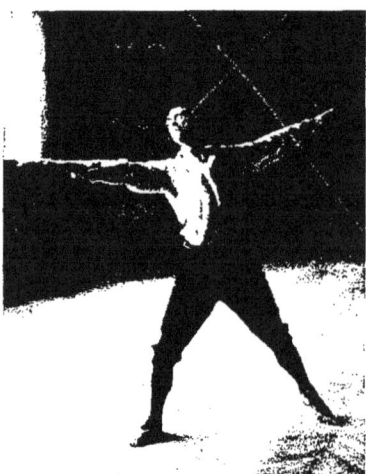

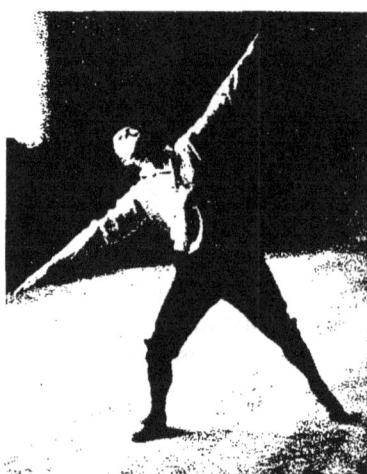

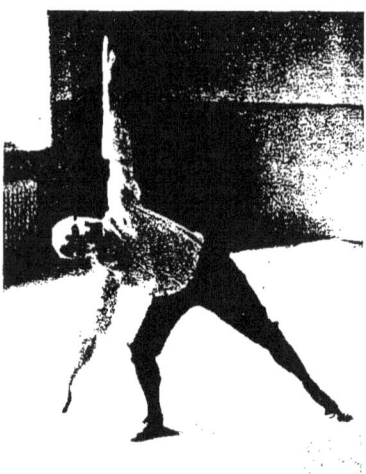

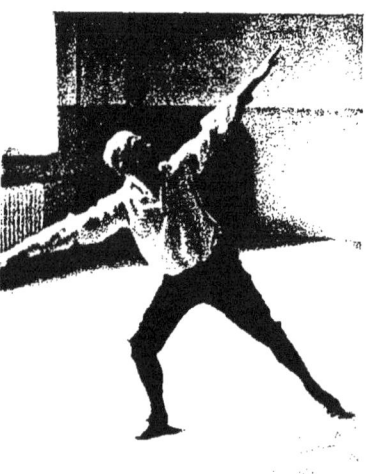

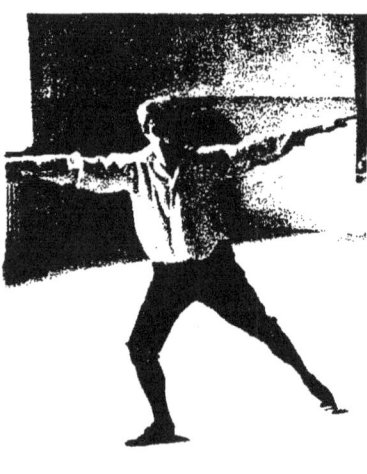

70

The great Vertical
(See Plate 28)

Another movement-picture arises if the student does not allow himself to be drawn forward by the goal and led into an urgent lunge, an exaggerated step forward, - but, emphasizing his vertical stature in height and the direction-finding force, he moves towards the goal.

In the previous movement-picture, the body was transformed into a balance, which swung as far as the vertical; now it becomes height and swings to the horizontal.

The student prepares for a step and moves one arm forward towards the goal and then to height; at the same time, he enhances height to the utmost. Gradually taking a firmer foothold and with growing tension, he leads height back again into the forward-seeking horizontal. The other arm is pointing downward.* Then the bodily tension is released, while simultaneously the free foot comes forward and the arm is lowered, so that a new step may be begun.

An enhancement of this movement, carrying height into the forward horizontal, comes about when not only the arm but the whole upright body moves and grows into the horizontal, pointing to the goal. Just as the arrow lies on the stretched string and is imbued with the power of direction, so now the student holds himself poised in balance upon the supporting leg, which is bent low. The free leg and arm point backward, relaxed; the line of vision and the line passing through arm and trunk go directly to the forward aim.

Then height is erected once more, beginning slowly to relax; the gradual relaxation is completed when the arm sinks to rest. The free leg finished the step and makes for another one.**

In this first enhancement, the eyes remain constantly fixed on the goal. If, however, as he rises from the poised span in the horizontal, the student lets the goal move up, from the horizontal to the zenith, and follows the arc of its path with eyes and body, he will come through a low backward bend, again into the horizontal,* and will have passed through the whole semi-circle. Again there arises a great sustaining tension, carried only upon the ball of the foot. Height is thus carried through the horizontal and brought back to height again.** It is a most difficult test of balance. The student must be held and carried by the line of sight directed to the goal, by his constant awareness of height and his confidence in its forces.

There is always a danger that this movement will become empty. To keep it in rhythmic flow, to let the breathing flow freely through it, and with determination to make the line of sight always precede the movement - all this, as well as keeping one's balance, demands great concentration and a consciousness of space and direction permeating the whole body.

Something fundamentally new marks this stage of gymnastic education. In the lower school, movement is a unity; it simply arises out of the instinct to move in a rhythm natural to breathing and blood circulation and is mirrored in consciousness by the head. The body lives and expresses itself through the will.

---

* The arm hangs down, loosely and naturally.
** With this, the other arm comes forward and is laid in the horizontal, pointing towards the goal.
* The arm which is otherwise inactive, is lifted forward, so that both arms together represent the balance; both hands with palms upward would be like the scale-pans. Bothmer often did this without the participation of the second arm, but from one of his sketches it is clear that he also thought of the balance as being made by the two arms.
** This happens with feet remaining in the same position; it is not connected with a change of feet, as might appear to be the case from the pictures.

Plate 28 – The great Vertical

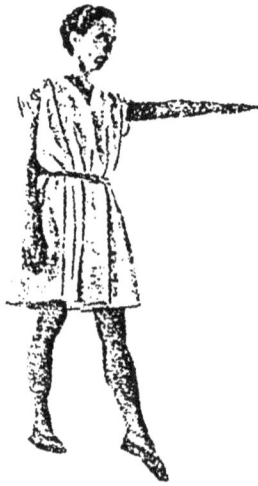

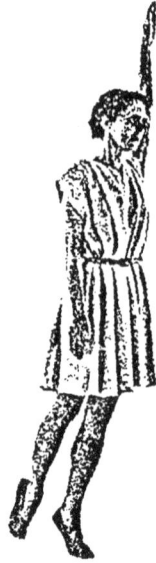

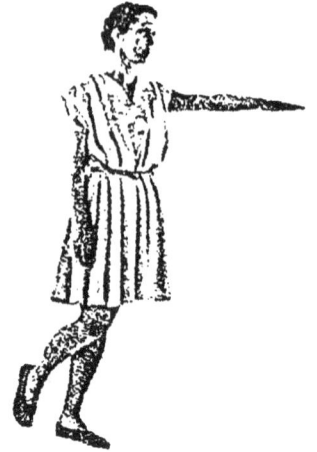

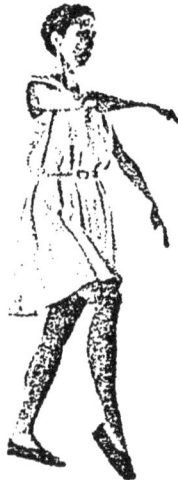

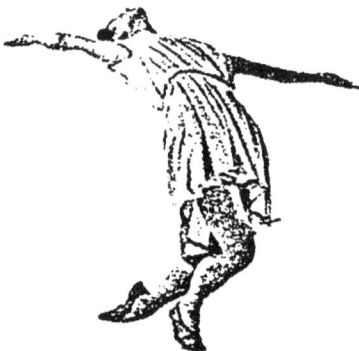

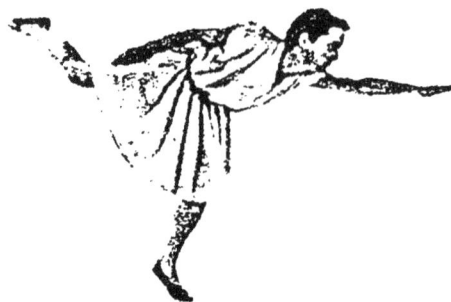

There is always a danger that this movement will become empty. To keep it in rhythmic flow, to let the breathing flow freely through it, and with determination to make the line of sight always precede the movement - all this, as well as keeping one's balance, demands great concentration and a consciousness of space and direction permeating the whole body.

Something fundamentally new marks this stage of gymnastic education. In the lower school, movement is a unity; it simply arises out of the instinct to move in a rhythm natural to breathing and blood circulation and is mirrored in consciousness by the head. The body lives and expresses itself through the will.

In the upper school it is consciousness which dominates; the limb-system conforms to conscious aims and intentions. Rhythm, and above all the rhythm of breathing, swings more and more freely over the movement. The step becomes the measure of the movement.

The very evident geometrical character of the exercises in the lower school recedes in the middle school, to appear again in the upper school in quite a new form, - in conscious awareness, through the dimensions and their interweaving, of the infinitudes of space, and of the great spherical movements.

In the exercises just described, horizontal swings to vertical, vertical to horizontal, without losing their respective qualities - given to them by the gymnast - of width and height, horizontal and vertical. Such interpretations are repeated and enhanced in the upper school. They summon the consciousness to greater activity.

Walking or stepping can also serve movement which are not so evidently dominated by a goal in space, but where the idea of an aim or goal only lights up at some essential moment. This already happened, though less noticeably, in the rhythm of the two interlacing circles behind the back, and then, a little more strongly, in the upward rise after the activated fall.

Walking or stepping can also serve movements which are not so evidently dominated by a goal in space, but where the idea of an aim or goal only lights up at some essential moment. This already happened, though less noticeably, in the rhythm of the two interlacing circles behind the back, and then, a little more strongly, in the upward rise after the activated fall.

The two following exercises, - related and yet diametrically opposed, - have the same critical moment in their rhythm when the goal becomes important for the gymnast and demands to be comprehended in full consciousness.

Distorted Height

(See Plate 29)

The foot prepares for a step, while height is emphasized by raised arms.* (33) The arms lead the body up in flowing movement, as high as possible, and then roll it in a far-reaching movement forward and downward into a spiral, sweeping right round until they are vertical again, with the head pressed down into the center of the spiral. The hands now take the place of the head and look forward. It is a distortion of height, with loss of human stature, - a dead point.

Now, out of a new resolve, the gymnast follows the upward-pointing force of the arms and tries to straighten up. Feeling the way upward with his hands, he comes from below into a distorted width, which lies like a horizontal yoke upon his neck, - another moment of frustration.

Trying to pass through the horizontal, he makes yet another resolve, and this time turns the horizontal about its own axis. Now the head can rise again; eyes find the goal, the supporting foot comes fully to the ground, while the other is free to take a step, and the arms, released, can raise the gymnast to height once more. In a renewed enhancement of height, the rhythm begins again.

In a dramatic event, at times breath-taking, and full of strong tensions and restricted movements, amounting almost to negation of the human form and leading twice to moments when the movement comes to nothing; first, as though caught in a snail-shell, from which only the feelers poke out, and then when height is split beneath the yoke of the horizontal. So much the greater is the release when it comes. Turning the horizontal in its axis through 360 degrees brings freedom to the human form and to human movement and gives the possibility of taking another step.

Distorted Width

(See Plate 30)

If now the beam of the cross, turned upward with the freedom of potential activity, is turned back again in its axis through 180 degrees, the movement picture will alter fundamentally; it will not simply unroll in reverse.

The turning movement forces the head under the horizontal yoke again and with it the whole form, which has to bend low, while the arms as they lead downward make a small circle by joining the knuckles of the two hands closely, almost as though to form a suture and make an organic whole.

This little circle, derived from the horizontal, closes hard by the foot of the supporting leg; its center is the head, bent low.

The free leg has slipped far back.

---

* The palms of the hands, which faced one another as the arms were lifted sideways from the horizontal to the vertical, are then turned to face forward during the enhancement of height.

Plate 29 – Distorted height

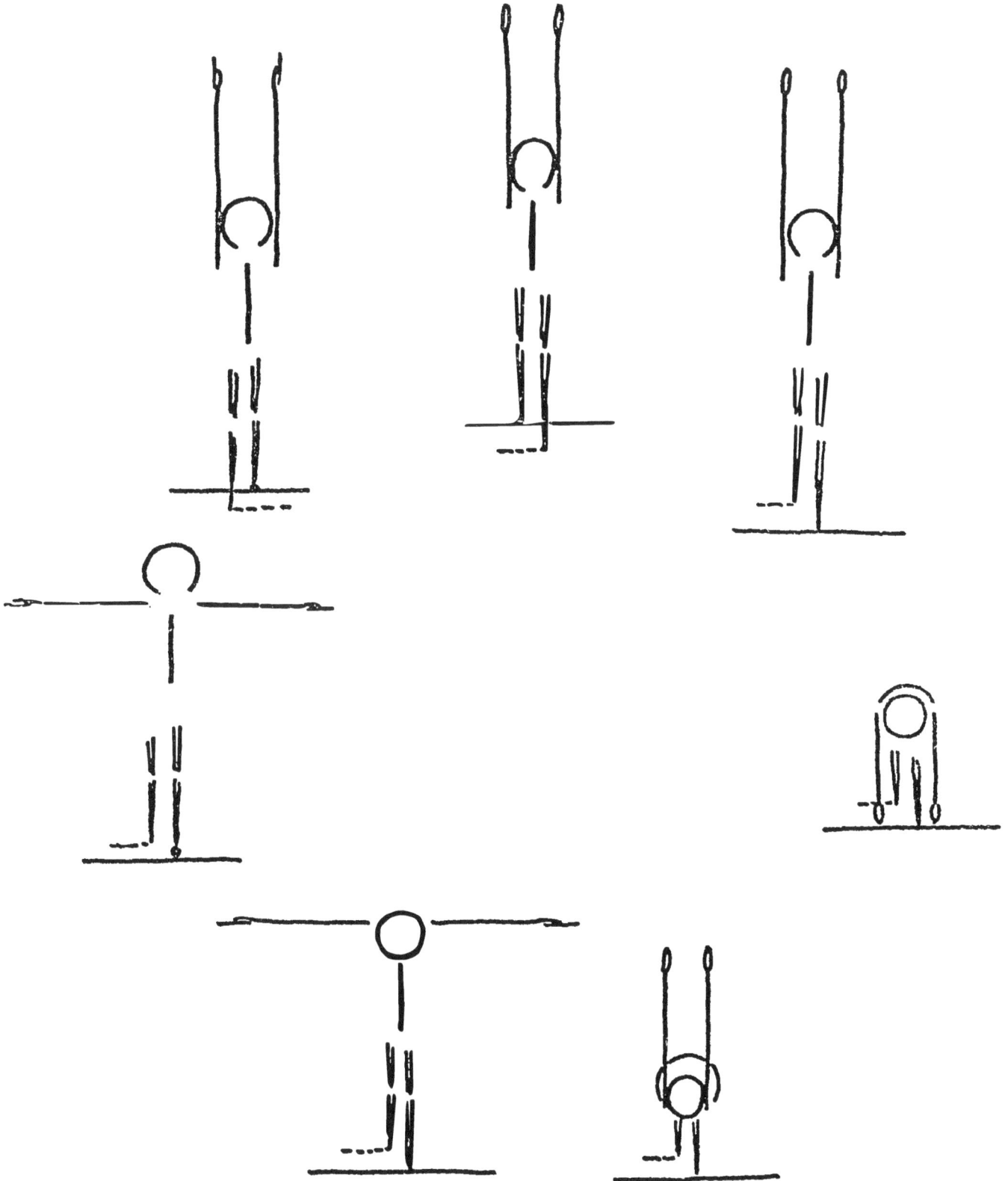

Plate 30 – Distorted width

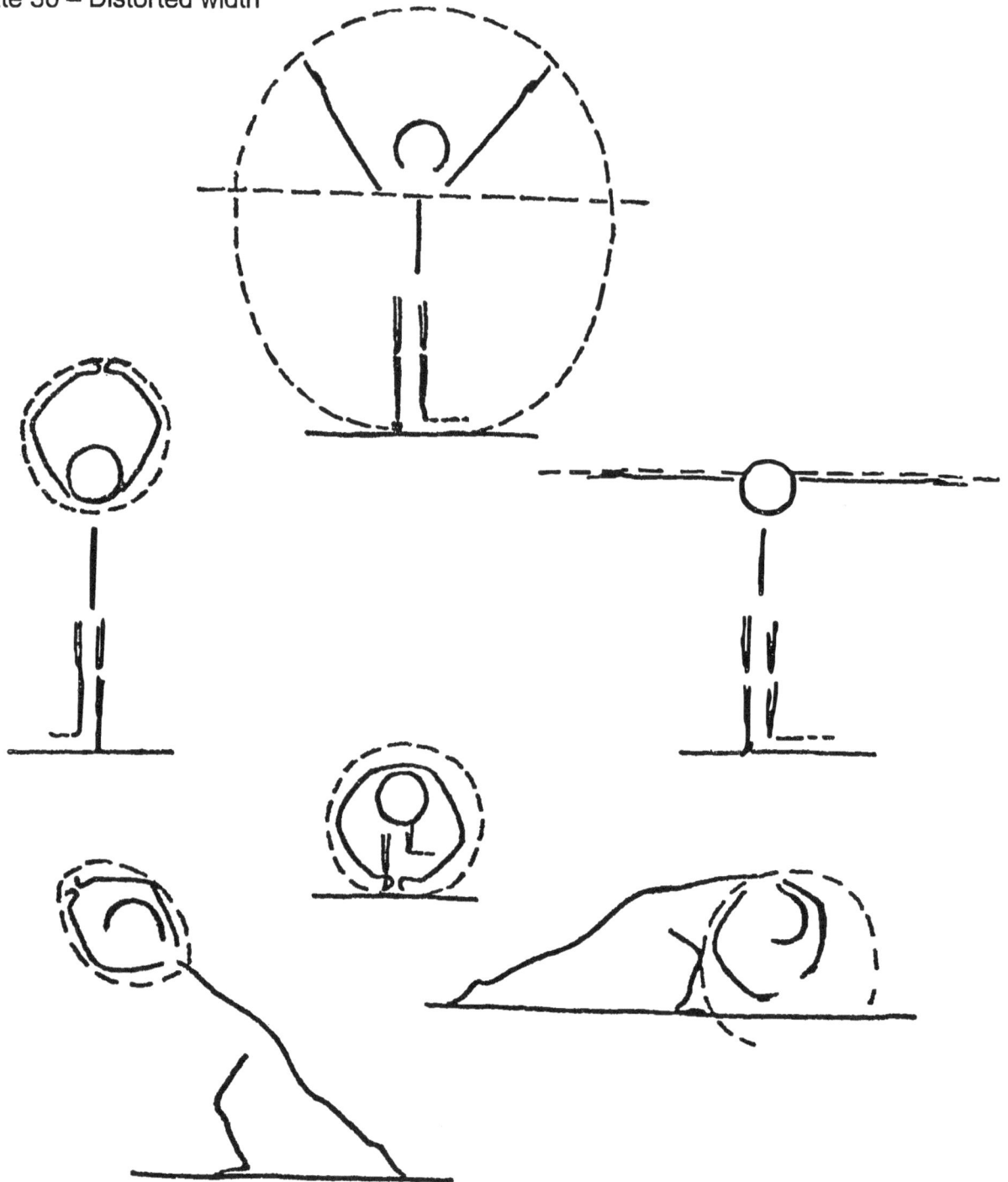

Now the gymnast carries the small circle of the arms to height and draws himself upright again; the free leg follows behind. In the last stage of rising upright, the head is lifted, the eyes hold fast to the goal and the little circle turns and opens upward, radiating out again to heights and widths. The free foot comes to the ground in front and the supporting leg is released, beginning at once to slide back again as the horizontal begins to turn once more about its axis.

With this, a larger circle - a circle without bodily form - arises. It had already commenced when the little circle, reaching the vertical, opened out; now it turns inside-out as it passes through the horizontal in width, closing with and in the little circle, in order to go with it through the lowest point.

Here below, the large circle releases the small one, in the center of which is the head, letting it go its own way back from depth to height. In the heights the small circle, now vertical, opens up into the large one as the eyes look forward, and then grows out into width, reaching the horizontal once more. As the circle opens upward, the center rays out into the large circle, as it closes downward, it is irradiated from without. The horizontally expanded with, turning in its axis, is the moment that divides the two. The release is great when, risen, the circle opens out again into the widths of space.

As these movements run their dramatic course, - and indeed in all exercises in which movement evolves in true gymnastic sequence, - space reveals man, and man reveals space. Movement which is freed by the infinitudes of space, on contrast to restricted, pent-up movement, brings to revelation the greater man who will incarnate in space and whose forces and rhythms guide the path of this gymnastic work.

Three Circles

(See Plate 31)

The rhythm of three circles, closing and opening with one another is a final enhancement and metamorphosis of the circling movement which, described earlier, was developed from the dynamic of the circle. The rhythmical conclusion of the swinging, circling movement sideways was a low bend. This bend need not always be part of a whole sequence of movements, but may arise and proceed in its own rhythm. The gymnast, standing, sets one foot sideways and, leaning to this side, reaches out widely with both arms, then closing them to a small circle around the head. As the body straightens up, the circle of the arms opens out again and the rhythm repeats to the other side.

In the bend, the whole body, led by the outer arm, strives to become rounded sideways to a large circle, which is poised and held in balance on the outer foot, set sideways. The inner foot lightly helps in buttressing the weight; the head moves into the center. The large circle formed by the outer arm, gives birth to the smaller one and sustains it. A third circle arises in between, almost unnoticed, as the large circle moves into the smaller one, and then again during the release to the standing position. The small circle comes to manifestation physically, the large one only partially and the middle one lives purely in the movement.

Plate 31

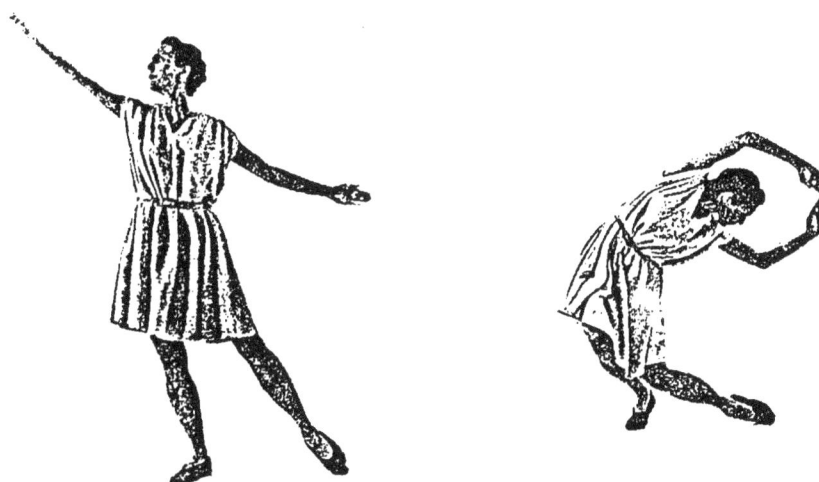

Circling about an inclined axis

(See Plate 32)

The fall through over-reaching into height was, in the repetition, changed in two directions, as has been described; through congestion of the movement, it took on a violent form, loaded with physical force; while through emphasis on the moving element, it was transformed into a milder, more rhythmical movement. The two variations were then brought together in a common form and a quiet rhythm.

Now the motif of the fall comes again in the upper school. This time, out of a new dynamic it leads to a new solution. Again the movement starts from height, to which the gymnast has raised himself after the pivotal turn. Raising up, he stands firmly on the supporting leg, while the free foot comes forward to prepare for a step.

Now he falls forward resolutely, setting height free and landing resiliently on the forward foot, wide and quiet in the cross of the inclined plane. The arms cross over and swing through depth out to width. The free leg moves backward to make room for the movement.

In the quiet flow of this swing into space, the movement no longer asks for the sudden turn which hitherto always followed the fall. This swinging fall comes to rest in the inclined plane, the two axis spread out in it in a cross. The eyes are directed forward to the goal.

Now, with a new resolve, the gymnast turns the cross; he makes the horizontal axis circle around in the inclined vertical one, keeping at right angles to it, while he holds firm and fast with the point of the free foot and with his line of sight.

The cross now lies on its back in the inclined plane and looks upward.

To reach height in vertical stature once more, the inclined axis bends backward as though to a circle, and is then led by the outspread arms through depth again to height.

While still upright, the gymnast had prepared for a step; then the turn on the supporting leg took place, for which the free leg had receded backward; now, in the rise following the turn, this leg becomes the supporting one. The long step backward is thus picked up again and with the completion of the step, height is regained.

This exercise has a flowing rhythm, wide and free, like breathing. It is confidence in the wide infinite span and in its courageous circling movement around height - the inclined vertical axis, - which brings mastery over the difficulty of balance. The wide expanse sustains us.*

The path of gymnastic education through the school years until the age of 18, has been given in a series of exercises, of which each represents a stage in itself. Experience has shown that no gap is to be felt in the sequence, and no pupil found them too easy.

A separate section will be devoted to jumping.

Viewed externally, what follows is ridiculously simple; the pupil can make all or nothing of it. Until now, the force of the will have been engaged predominantly in meeting and overcoming the resistance of the body, - of weight. Now the will-forces are called to great exertion in the pupil's consciousness. Just as the play of the hands of a clock would have no meaning for us, were it not that we are conscious of the being of "Time"; so now, in the exercises which follow for the upper school, the movements of the limbs would have no meaning, but for the pupils' consciousness of the great being "Space". The successive movements, even those which are yet to come, are pres-

---

* Bothmer did this exercise, like the last, with only one repetition; this accords with their form.

ent to the thinking consciousness as unembodied forms in space. Their time-rhythm is present to the hearing consciousness.

The pupil cannot quite bring this being of Space and Time to visible expression, but he can himself penetrate to an even deeper experience of it and give some idea of it in his movement.

Plate 32 – Circling about an inclined axis

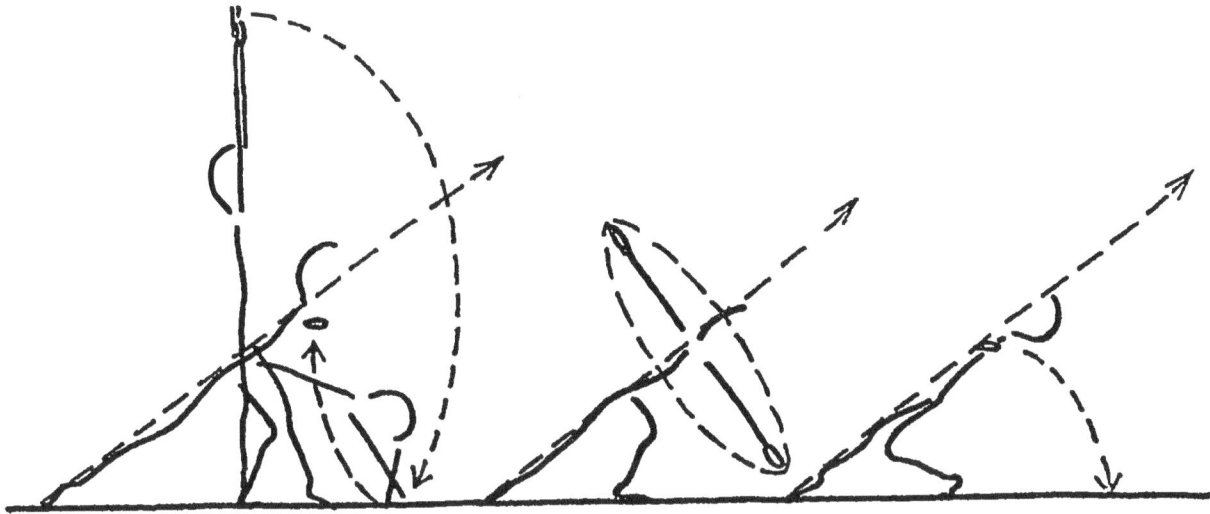

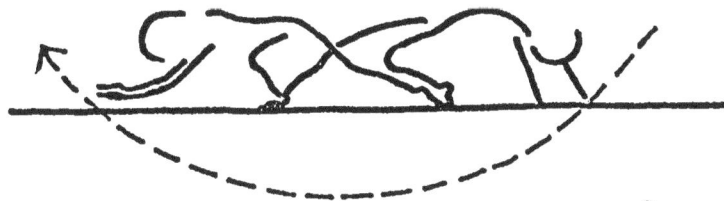

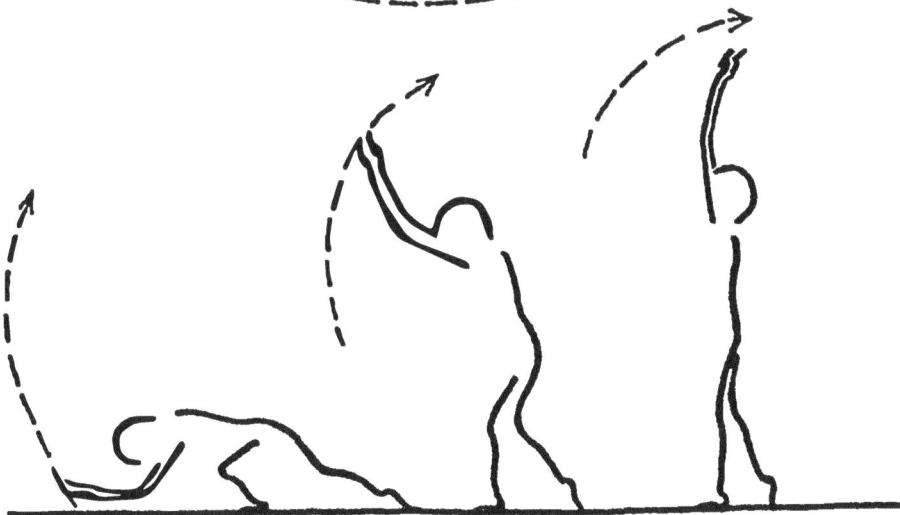

Dome of Crossed Arches

(See Plate 33)

Every time the gymnast moves his arms to and from height, he creates a half-circle above his head and reproduces the rounded form of the skull. To the forces which envelop the human form, sphere upon sphere, he tries to give definite spatial and rhythmical expression.

Over the simple cross of the vertical and horizontal, he builds spherical curves, arches. He lifts the arms to height and turning, first to the right and then to the left, he lets height grow from the apical point into the widths. Then facing forward again, he builds over these two arches a third and still greater arch. All the while the feet hold the direction to height firmly and carry the body poised in space.

The semicircles form a widely spanned dome over the horizontal plane of the outspread arms, one arch flung higher than the last; one blossoming out of the other to greater and greater heights and widths. After the last and highest span, the pupil turns and looks forward, arms in the balance of the horizontal; then he releases himself into the equilibrium of the "I stand upright, firmly on the ground, conscious of the dimension of space and of its over-arching forces."

The rhythm almost completely disappears into the growing, forming spaces. Space breathes. If, in spite of the great tension and the long awaited resolution, the gymnast can continue to breathe freely throughout the movement, space will become a second and greater breathing. Then the tensions will not be rigid, for the flow of breathing will keep them relaxed.

With the three semicircular arcs, accompanied by the turning of the body, the three mutually perpendicular planes have arisen:

> one dividing forward and backward,
> one dividing left and right
> one dividing above and below.

Meanwhile the direction towards the goal firmly held on the foundation-point established by the feet.

Plate 33

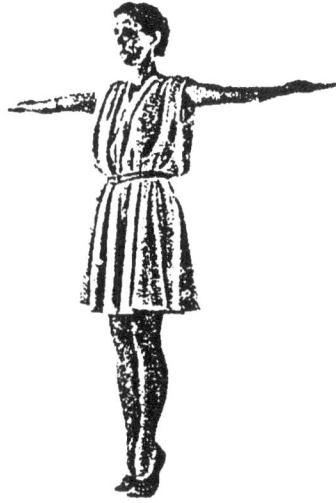

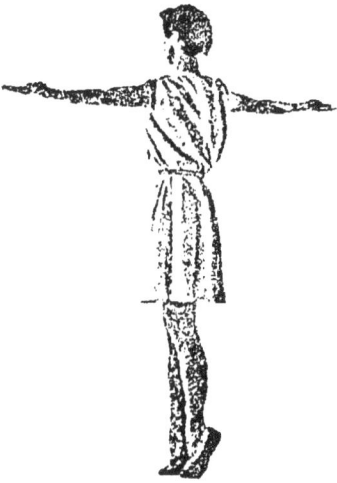

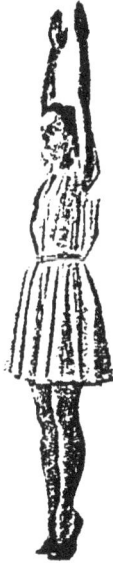

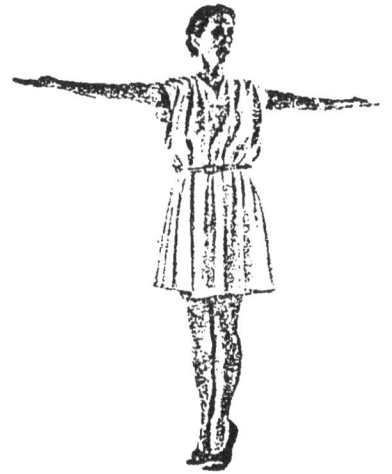

The Cross

(See Plate 34)

Even this point can be given freedom in that the gymnast, while measuring out the three dimensional planes and axis space, moves with forward and backward step.

First he unfolds the three dimensions of space, then one by one he takes them back again, bringing the one dimension inwardly into the other, till in the upright and widely spanned cross of man's stature, into which space with all its forces flows, the utmost interpenetration is attained. In the point - in the "I stand" - Space reaches final condensation, even it annuls itself, and in its stead stands conscious Man - one in the trinity of his inner powers: Thinking, Feeling and Willing. It is the greater Man - Man, the Measure of all Things.

I lay my arms in the forward direction and take a step forward;

I turn my hands palms upward and take the step back again;

I open my arms to width and take another step back;

I close my arms to height* and bend low to depth; my free leg receding to give room to the movement;

Then I rise up again to height; the free leg returning;

I carry height into width. My free foot comes forward full on the ground.

I carry the width, now permeated by height, forward; fasten my eyes on the goal and close the step;

I place the width, looking forward as it is and filled with height, into the resistance of the earth, into the point from which I took my start;

I release myself from spatial tension. The dimensions of space, interpenetrating one another and me, live on in my consciousness as powers of will.

I stand.

---

* In height, palms are turned forward.

Plate 34 – The cross

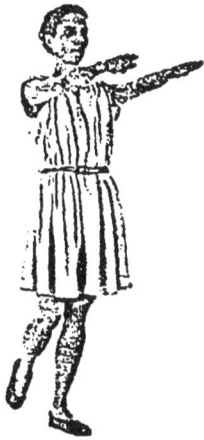

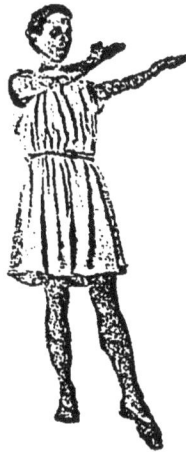

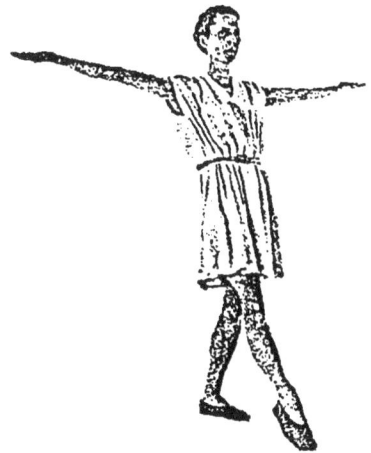

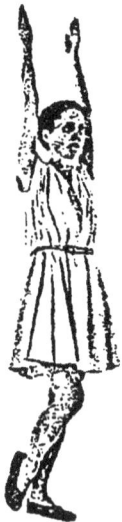

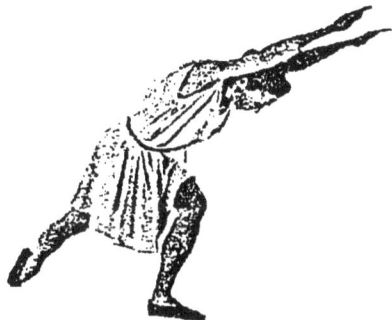

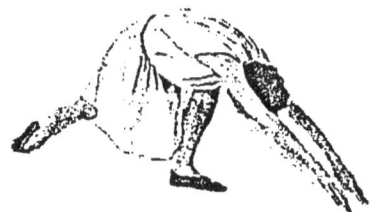

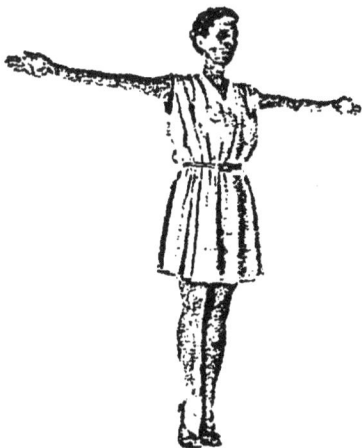

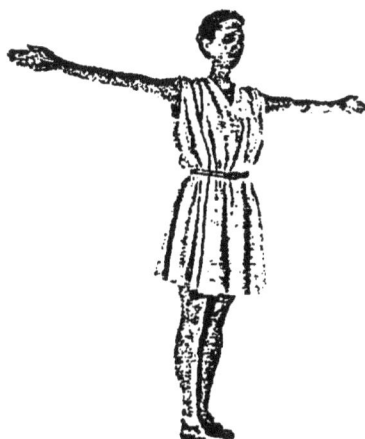

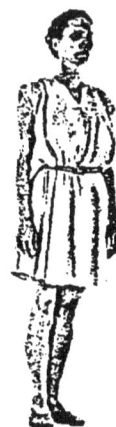

Walking, Running and Leaping

The best practice for walking is surely running, and for running, leaping. Plenty of, leaping, in various rhythms and in pairs or chains, encourages mobility, fires the will and has a formative effect.

In this method of gymnastic education, walking, running and leaping first occurred in the roundelays:

> "I stand,
> I walk, ...
> I run o'er the ground...
> I leap, I leap,
> And halt without sound."

It was the natural way to make the transition from standing to moving forward, which was enhanced and then slowed down again to standing. In standing, the child experiences his vertical stature and the resistance of the earth; in walking he feels the beat and measure of movement; the rhythm of running, he experiences as flowing movement, arising out of a natural interplay of forces; and in leaping he feels determined strength. A child at play runs gracefully, and it is all the better if the running is made into a game; but the game should contain some rhythm, perhaps given in words which he can say himself, such as "I run o'er the ground".

Running together in chains or in twos and threes, is a sociable exercise and of great value, for it helps children to learn to adjust and co-ordinate their own movements to those of others.

If running is really to be enjoyed, there must be a free interplay of forces. To allow the deeper breathing to stream freely through the movement, the vertical position proper to walking must be abandoned and the whole body, with its movement, must be rounded. The less the upper part of the body, (chest, arms and head) is stemmed against the movement, the freer and more joyful will running be. Head and arms should adapt themselves to the light, easy movement of the trunk.

Running is often enough only a sort of falling forward, with the legs trying to catch up. In gymnastic running, the play of forces should be lead and controlled at every step of the runner. The breathing takes care of the unity of the movement, flowing through it, ample and deep. In time, every step becomes a footing deliberately reaching out towards the goal. The foot not only catches up the fall; it feels and touches the earth. With the other foot, the runner springs off the resisting earth, resolving the tension in the free return of the leg. Running is essentially a reaching out into space; the runner ought to feel this.

Below, in the step, running is a raying, direction-giving force; above, it is circling force. The two interpenetrate. The pupil's attention should be turned sometimes more to one aspect, or to the other, until at least he perceives the interpenetration and masters it.

The circular rhythm of running may be developed through running itself; but it can arise from standing, though this is more difficult. The pupil stands completely relaxed and lifts his arms, loose to the fingertips, forward and upward; he moves them on, circling, as though stroking the surface of a sphere. It is as though he enveloped himself in this circling force, which, moving over the shoulder-blades and the back, can for a moment be felt almost physically, before it dives back into the rhythm again.

In the moment, when, coming from height, the circling rhythm takes hold of the body, the pupil resolves the movement as though with a soft touch, breaking into a light and easy running step. During the run, the rhythm of the circle closes upward again and with this the movement ends as gradually as it began. With practice, this way of running instills into the run an unusually rhythmical force which then has its effect on all running. It is more easily derived from walking than from standing.

It is really the highest degree of lightness - of anti-gravitational force, - overcoming gravity, which can be called up in running. The pupil feels drawn forward by the movement. Running itself becomes a rhythm.

Such an exercise requires the mature forces of the human being in thinking, feeling and willing. Until such time as this is possible, the example of the teacher is all that is needed. This way of running perhaps comes nearest to that of the young child, unconscious in his movements, whose graceful play still has a touch of heaven

The First Leap

The running step may from time to time be enhanced to a leap, long and high in the air. Ever anew, this stimulates the reaching forward into space. The leap is to begin with only a rather higher and more springy running step, such as comes in the roundelay for the small children:

"I leap, I leap, I leap ..."

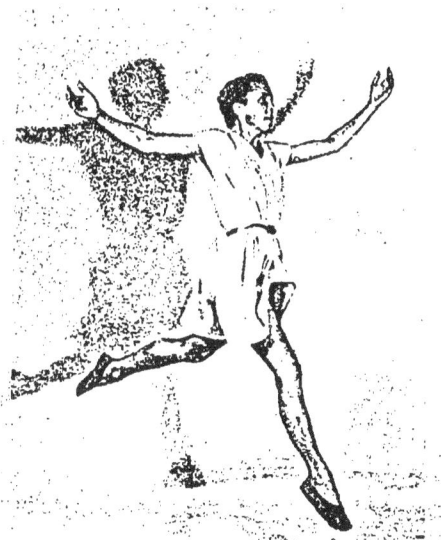

These running leaps are particularly good in bringing consciousness to the feet as they aim forward, touching and feeling for the ground, like a hand. This kind of awareness in the foot, lends grace and vigor to the running of a grown man. The jump can be repeated rhythmically in running, as follows:

"Run, run, leap; run, run, leap..."

or

"Short, short, long..."

or

"ta ta tam, ta ta tam..."

Only in this rhythm will the leap come to its expression; it will be a jump of joy. This goes well, done in pairs or in long lines. If done singly, the peculiar nature of this rhythmic run and leap requires the fire and strength of the whole human being. It can be enhanced if the pupil, holding a staff horizontally at center of gravity, swings it vertically up and catches it again. In following the staff, which he swings high with a long arm as he leaps, the pupil emphasizes the forward and up-ward-leading power of the leap.

A difficult enhancement and enrichment of this rhythm comes about if the leap is carried upward and gives wings by swinging both arms upward from width height, and is then caught again by the outspread arms in both these forms, the leap is full of radiating form.

In the rhythm "Short, short, long", the leap up by itself is a valuable exercise. If it is practiced alone, the arm circling as though stroking the surface of a sphere, catches up the movement as it falls and leads it up again to height until a position of balance has been achieved, alighting on the foot which led the leap. This way of catching the descent from the leap and raising the movement up to the vertical again is similar to the rise after the turn following the fall into the inclined plane.

The Second Leap

While the rhythm "short, short, long" finds natural expression in a forward movement, in "short, long" the ? movement is at first held and then rises steeply to height "Ga - llop, ga - llop, ga - llop..."

The body is drawn together in this leap and becomes a ball. In the descent this tension is released again into the vertical with the intermediate step.

The spring is best begun from the standing position by treading backwards; it should either be done lightly and quickly, (as the sound of the word "gallop" in German would indicate), or it can be done very powerfully, swinging the outstretched arms in circles, with clenched fists.

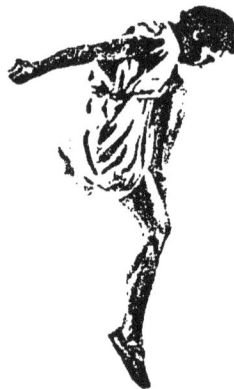

The galloping leap should always end in running, in order gradually to quiet the pulse and the breathing. The transition from galloping to running brings a strong sense of the difference between movement which is held back, and movement which is given free rein. The force in this leap is all gathered inward.

The single leap, "short, long", without rhythmic repetition, can also be practiced in two forms. Either it may be done with the body drawn together, accompanied by the circling arms, which flinging upward, emphasize the descent and pull the body erect again as the foot comes strongly to the ground. The over-reaching movement which results must be immediately relaxed, otherwise the movement will lead to the fall into the inclined plane. Or the spring is done lightly, with the body erect and with outspread arms; the arms then simply hold the balance, and the descent is caught up with a light, flexible step. This variation may be done backwards by driving the leap from a forward step. The accompanying words would be:

> "ta - tam - tata"

in which "ta" is the contraction before the take-off.

The Third Leap

The rhythm arises of its own accord, when the galloping leap is practiced by itself. The inner dynamic of this rhythm can however be enhanced into a second leap. This new rhythm comprises two leaps, using alternate feet.[*] (36) The last leap ends directly in the point in which the gymnast finds his balance when the rhythm comes to rest.

> "ta - tam - tata - tam - ta".

At the end, the gymnast stands on one leg, the other held free, arms outspread and eyes upon the goal.

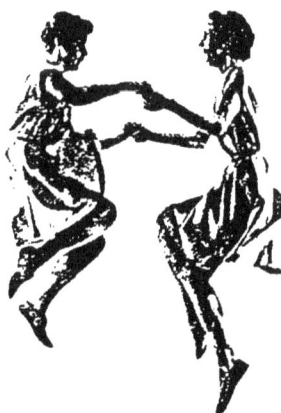

It is characteristic of this rhythm that it unites with the widths and can only be done with arms in the horizontal or circling closely around it.

The first leap, "short, short, long; short, short, long..." was accompanied by a swing of the arms from width to height and back to width; the second leap, "short, long; short, long..." by arms circling

---

[*] Bothmer regarded this leap as a union of the two preceding single rhythms: followed by the catching up movement which brings it to a close.

from depth to height, and back to depth; the third, "short, long, short, short, long, long", is done with arms in the horizontal. This reveals the true character of the three rhythms. The first belongs to height and is filled with raying forces; the second belongs to depth, with rounding and enclosing forces; the third belongs to the middle, the balance between height and depth. Raying force above, rounded below, this leap is vertical. The third rhythm may also be done with a backward leap; it is therefore possible to do it in pairs. Two stand opposite one another and, taking one another by both hands, they leap together, one forward and the other backward. Then "You and I" stand face to face once more, as in the first roundelay.

The gradual enhancement of this leaping exercise, as it has been described is:

> "ta - tam - tata,
>
> ta - tam - tata,
>
> ta - tam - tata - tam - ta"

It can be done repeatedly, forward or backward or alternating, simply or in pairs, and is a very good exercise in rhythm, bringing the leaps to a fine conclusion.

It is not to be recommended that either teacher or pupil should count to the rhythms; they should rather be apprehended with the musical ear, followed and then tested down to the finest detail of movement.

These ways of leaping take the whole human being into account; they also avoid over-exuberance in movement, which is ungymnastic and distorts the picture of man. After all, the training of walking, running and leaping must also be guided by the form of man and the true balance of his forces. As a part of gymnastic education, this training leads to the same conclusion as the whole; after the last leap, the human being comes to rest at a point on the ground and finds his true balance between width and height and goal. Then he releases the outward span, but lets space and the springing force work on within him.

"I stand, spanned into space, holding my balance and conscious of the springing forces within me.

Running and leaping may be enriched with the help of staff or spear; leaping may be accompanied by the tambourine and the cymbals, the accented beat always being given to the highest point of the leap.

In running, staff and spear, resting in the palm of the hand, are held high, pointing forward horizontally with the arm slightly bent. During the run, the spear may also be thrown upward and caught again, keeping it horizontal. This too can be enhanced to a leap and repeated in the rhythm: "ta - tam - tata - tam - ta": The gymnast throws the spear up horizontally at the first leap; as it returns from height he catches it with the second leap and comes simultaneously to the standing position, with the spear pointing forward, high in one hand, the other arm raised sideways, holding his balance on one foot.

Afterword

The gymnastic education here described is rigorous schooling, engaging the human being to the full. For the teacher, it is an inexhaustible source of inspiration, providing a wide field of gymnastic activity.

Teacher, as well as pupil, in the course of his own work, will be able to conclude from the totality of every movement-picture, - from the very idea of the exercise, - what each single element of the movement should be; and in working at the movements, he will mould and form them, and through them, himself. The fact that every single part must have its proper and meaningful place in the gymnastic idea as a whole, or can be derived therefrom, will ensure the wakeful participation of the mind and spirit in the external events which befall the body. The conviction will grow that such a sequence of gymnastic exercises, both in the detail and in the whole, is the beginning of a quite new edifice of bodily training and education, the further wise development of which will be stimulated.

In the Waldorf School in Stuttgart, this gymnastic education went hand in hand with the education by means of eurythmy, given by Dr. Rudolf Steiner, which brings the being of the spoken word and of music to expression in bodily movement as "visible speech" and "visible song". Eurythmy, as a school of movement, influences the development of the human being mainly through the soul; gymnastics mainly through the body.

That both these should be used simultaneously in the education of boys and girls together, appears to the author to be the ideal. They guard against and resolve the cramping psychological and physical condition which threaten even at an early age, making the young human being healthy and strong, happy in the consciousness that forces of a divine, spiritual origin are at work, forming him in body and soul.

Bothmer Exercises in the School Curriculum

Class III: First Roundelay. From far and wide we come "to build a house". Outside and inside meet in a dialogue: "You and I, I and you, seek one another, find one another". Light running and jumping movements form the main theme.

Class IV: Second Roundelay. The power of man's vertical stature transforms the "house" into a "tower". It is surrounded by storms and by the sound of the bells echoing into the widths of space. Based firmly on the ground, the heights reach out into the widths of space... "and still wider". To the movements of running and jumping is added rhythmical swinging.

Third Roundelay. Movement towards a goal is expressed by the two concentric circles which move in opposite directions. For a moment the two circles meet and the movement is enhanced. Vigorous steps are alternately longer and shorter.

Class V: Springing jumps give vitality especially by the early gymnastic exercises and bring out the contrasts: above and below, height and breadth, lightness and weight. (See: Play between Weight and Lightness. The triangle, The re-entrant triangle.)

Class VI: Rod exercises. The child experiences the rod's various qualities, - its roundness, its length and its strength. These exercises strengthen the upright, vertical stature in all its aspects from stretching lightly upward to standing firmly upon the ground. (See: The rolling rod, Triangle with rod, The Square).

Class VII: Swinging movements of the arms lead to an experience of center and periphery. The pupil experiences his vertical stature in a resilient up-and-down movement. Rhythm arises and planes are spanned. (See: Sideways circling, Spring into the center, Rhythm.)

Class VIII: Unison of spring and swing. Gravity is enhanced, the spring is activated and the swing modified. The rhythm of the preceding exercises is thus differentiated, - at one time more dramatic, at another more gay. Interplay of supporting leg and free leg. Sustained by the wide periphery, the human stature is experienced in outer space. (See: The Fall into Space.)

Class IX: Starting form the experience of gravity, spring and swing become thrusting and gliding movements. Out of this new polarity where the rhythmic element seems temporarily lost, walking and stepping movements arise and a new rhythm comes to life. In walking a new and threefold relation to the surrounding world is created. Space is now taken hold of from within. (See: Fall into the point. Rhythm of two interlacing circles, Waling with circling arms, Twofold eight.)

Class X: Exercises with an aim or goal. From the simple forward lunge and the backward throwing movement, these exercises in their further course lead to a quiet rising and falling movement, in the rhythm of which the power of balance finds expression. The line of sight becomes more independent. The rhythmically flowing movements grow quieter and a new uprightness is achieved, in unison with the consciously active line of sight. The pupil becomes aware of the essential form of the head. (See: Movement towards an aim or goal. The great horizontal, The great vertical.)

Class XI: The circle is formed from without, when through the inward tension of a spiral, movement has been directed to an aim or goal within. Finally, the whole human form enters into - even becomes - the circle, which is sustained from the periphery of space, and in which inner and outer meet. The realization of space here finds its culmination and all they rhythms to rest. (See: Distorted height, Distorted width, Three circles.)

Class XII: The human form is revealed in a threefold way in the concluding exercises. In quiet, circling movement, imbued at one and the same time with width and with clearly directed aim, human rhythms are united with the cosmic rhythms. One after another the gymnast experiences the three planes and emerges from their several realms. It is like drawing a deep breath. In the three-fold spiraling movement of "growing out over height into width", the dome arises, revealing the form of the head, an image of the vault of heaven. The horizontal plane becomes the sustaining ground.

The final exercise is filled with the radial, directing forces of the limb man. Working in unison, they bring forth the human form and stature, in which all the possibilities of movement come to rest as in a picture. (See: Circling about an inclined axis, Dome of crossed arches, The Cross.)

www.ingramcontent.com/pod-product-compliance
Lightning Source LLC
Chambersburg PA
CBHW081420270326

41931CB00015B/3349